The
Renal Diet
Cookbook for the
Newly Diagnosed

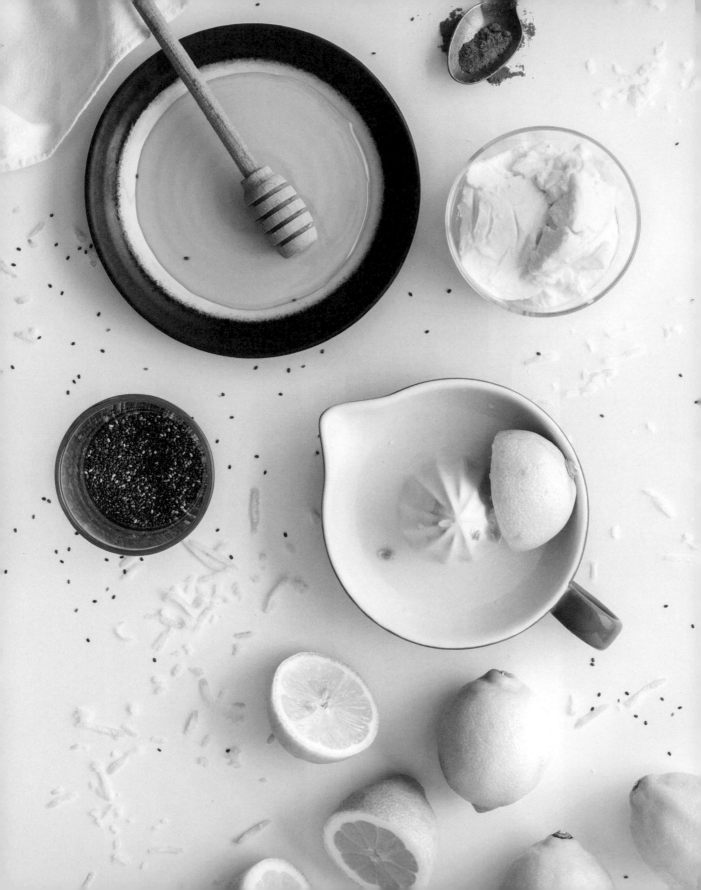

The Renal Diet Cookbook for the Newly Diagnosed

The Complete Guide to Managing Kidney Disease and Avoiding Dialysis

SUSAN ZOGHEIB, MHS, RD, LDN

Foreword by Jay Wish, MD

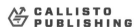

CALLISTO PUBLISHING

In memory of Dely Mateo

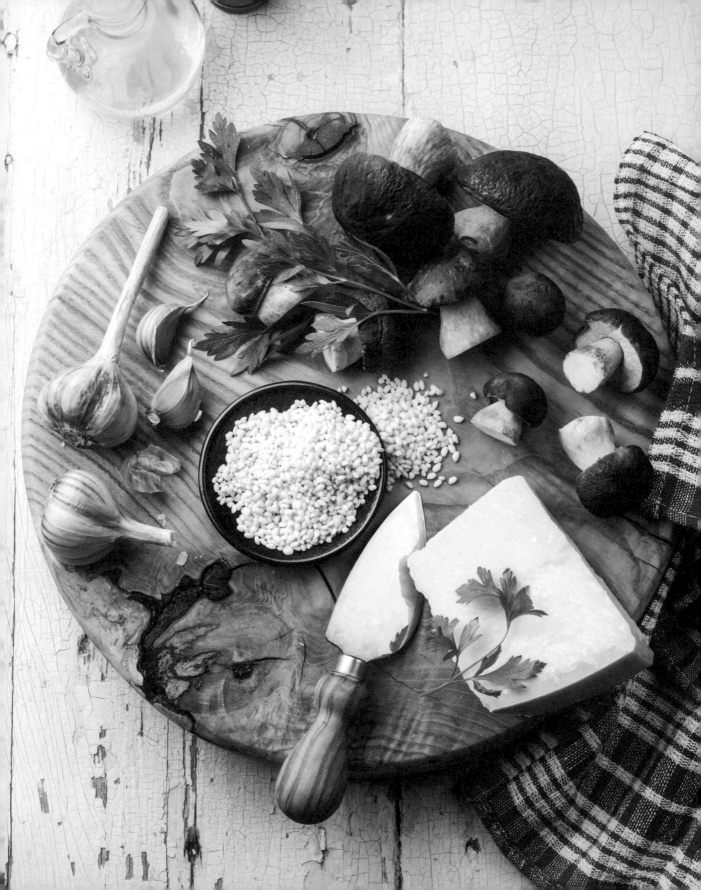

Contents

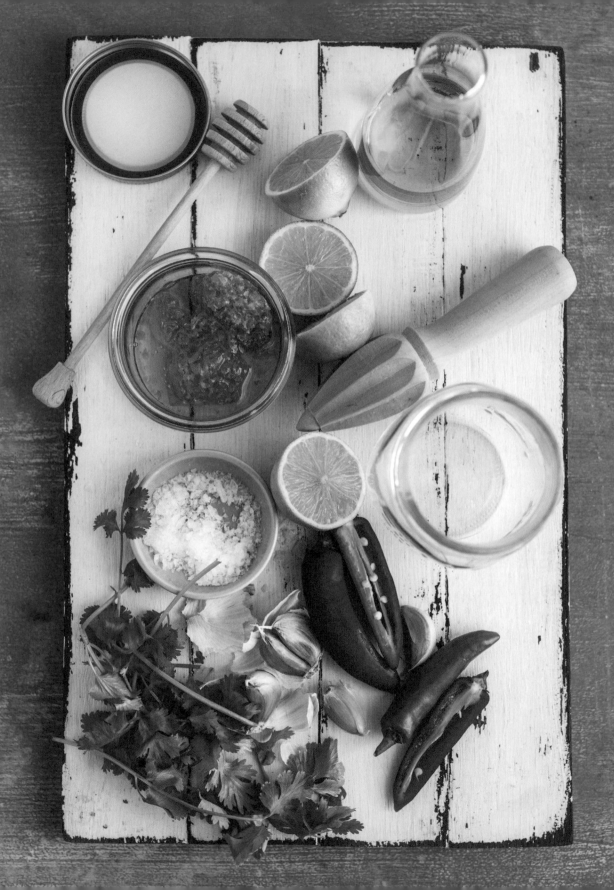

Foreword

Chronic kidney disease (CKD) affects over 30 million Americans, but fortunately, only a small fraction will progress to requiring dialysis or a kidney transplant. We've known for over 50 years that diet has a significant effect on the clinical outcome of patients with CKD by slowing the rate of disease progression, delaying the onset of symptoms, improving the internal environment of the body, and decreasing the risk of cardiovascular disease. For patients who also have cardiovascular disease, diabetes, high blood pressure, or high cholesterol levels, dietary treatment can go a long way not only to stabilize kidney function but to improve survival, too.

Unfortunately, learning to follow the renal diet, which is used to manage CKD by controlling one's intake of sodium, potassium, phosphorus, proteins and fluids, can be challenging for people who are newly diagnosed with CKD. The renal diet can feel even more daunting if patients have already been following a restrictive diet to reduce their intake of sugars (to manage diabetes) or fats (to manage high cholesterol levels). The obvious question that many patients with CKD have is this: "With so many restrictions in my diet, what is left for me to eat?" They fear that the renal diet will require them to eat bland, boring food, which can make healthy eating difficult and unsustainable.

Diet has a significant effect on the clinical outcome of patients with CKD

Thus, I welcome this new book by Susan Zogheib because it provides patients with CKD the tools they need to plan and prepare meals that are delicious yet within the dietary restrictions necessary for managing CKD successfully. The 4 weeks of daily menus provide ample variety for every taste, and the recipes she offers are delicious and feature wholesome yet affordable ingredients. The tips that accompany each recipe allow for substitutions to suit individual preferences or restrictions. The menus can appeal to the entire household of patients with CKD, too, so patients don't have to feel isolated by eating separate meals from their loved ones. By eating these delicious, well-balanced meals together, the entire family benefits.

Susan Zogheib is not only a highly-trained registered dietitian with extensive experience in the nutritional management of patients with CKD. She is also a creative chef who has collected delicious, kidney-friendly recipes over many years. She works directly with many different patients, so she knows which diets and meal plans work to maximize patient acceptance and sustainability. I have personally worked with Susan on many occasions to develop programs that help patients with CKD manage their blood phosphorus levels, and I am amazed by her knowledge, energy, and passion for improving the outcomes for this vulnerable population.

The Renal Diet Cookbook for the Newly Diagnosed is comprehensive in its scope. It explains the nature of CKD, provides rationale for the dietary restrictions required to manage CKD, and offers a complete toolkit for meal preparation, including shopping lists, menus, and recipe customization tips. The wide variety of delicious but healthy meals can help newly-diagnosed patients see that the renal diet is not a death knell for satisfying dishes and familiar flavors, but rather a tasty opportunity to explore a new way of eating that slows disease progression whilst renewing health and vigor. Susan's unique perspective as a renal dietitian and food expert makes this book an indispensable guide for the bewildering dietary challenges faced by patients who are learning to manage CKD, and I applaud her for addressing this unmet need.

Jay B. Wish, MD
Professor of Clinical Medicine
Division of Kidney Diseases
Indiana University School of Medicine
Indianapolis, IN

Introduction

Managing chronic kidney disease (CKD) requires lifestyle adjustments, but it might help to know you're not alone. In fact, over 31 million people in the United States are diagnosed with some malfunction of their kidneys or are battling kidney disease. As a registered dietitian (RD) with extensive experience assisting patients in taking control over their kidney disease, I have helped patients not only manage the physical symptoms associated with this disease but also cope with the emotional toll that this life change can take. Without knowing what the future holds, uncertainty, fear, depression, and anxiety can be common. It may even feel like dialysis is inevitable, and you may be asking yourself if it is worth the time or effort to try and manage this stage of the disease, or if it's even possible to delay the progression. As an expert in this field, I can assure you it is not just possible; it's yours to achieve—only 1 in 50 diagnosed with CKD end up on dialysis. So together, with the right tools, we can work to delay and ultimately prevent end-stage renal disease and dialysis. Success is earned through diet modifications and lifestyle changes. Using simple, manageable strategies, I have watched firsthand as my patients

Only 1 in 50 diagnosed with CKD end up on dialysis

empowered themselves with knowledge. They have gone on to lead full, productive, and happy lives, continuing to work, play, and enjoy spending time with their loved ones—just the way it should be!

Diet is a vital part of treatment for CKD, and it can help immensely in slowing the progression of the disease. There are ingredients that help the kidneys function, while others make the kidneys work harder. This book will focus on crowding out the unhealthy with the healthy and helpful. Also, targeting factors like salt and carbohydrate intake is important to reduce the risk of hypertension, diabetes, and other diseases that can result from kidney failure. I can't emphasize enough the importance of consulting a dietitian throughout the progression of CKD in order to optimize health, and this book is a good start, as it's designed specifically for the treatment of this population.

As an RD, I have years of firsthand experience treating patients at all stages of CKD. In this third book of my series, I want to give you, as a newly diagnosed individual, a better idea of how to manage these critical first stages with proper nutrition and recipes tailored to your unique condition. You may feel like you're in uncharted territory, and navigating your new dietary requirements can be challenging. At first, all of the new food dos and don'ts can be confusing, even frustrating, to you and your family. On top of that, it is common to be dealing with other health issues, such as hypertension or diabetes, which can add to the food restrictions.

This book is designed to help. With over 100 recipes, plus tips and tricks, this book can help us tackle your new challenge together. It describes exactly what you can eat and what you should try to avoid, and features unique meal plans that can be tailored to your needs and likes. It will also provide you with specific diet information, such as the types of fruit with lower potassium, or the dairy choice with lower phosphorus, so you'll understand the best options when you prepare meals and snacks.

In this time of change and uncertainty, the knowledge you gain from these pages will give you the power to take your life into your hands and make changes to benefit you in the short and long term. I hope to educate and inspire you with new, easy ways to change the trajectory of your health. Adopting a kidney-friendly lifestyle can be challenging at first, but following these recipes will reduce the anxiety associated with selecting smart food options for your everyday life. And lest you worry that your new diet is restrictive or unsustainable, I want to assure you that these recipes are both easy and delicious, and they will give you a realistic, satisfying way to make this lifestyle change. This book will guide you each step of the way. In doing so, it will help take the stress of meal planning out of the equation, and help you focus on the truly important things in life.

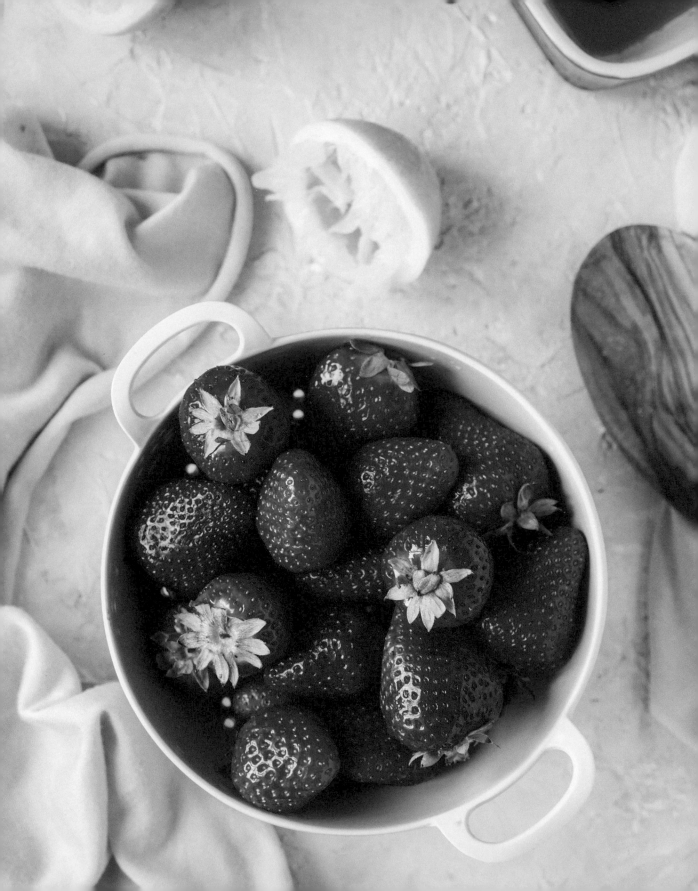

CHAPTER ONE

What You Need to Know About Kidney Disease

While a diagnosis of chronic kidney disease (CKD) may seem scary at first, and it's most likely leaving you with a lot of questions, it can be managed very effectively. It just requires a little bit of time, patience, and exploration, so you can see all the pieces of the big picture. The first step in managing kidney disease is understanding it. In this chapter, we'll review the vital role your kidneys play, what goes wrong when you develop kidney disease, and how diet plays an extremely important role in managing kidney disease.

What Does a CKD Diagnosis Mean?

During this hectic time of diagnosis and management of your new lifestyle, it is helpful to explore CKD and outline a few common symptoms. CKD can be defined simply as the gradual loss of kidney function. Since the body is constantly producing waste, the kidneys play a key role in removing these toxins and keeping your system functioning properly. Tests can be done to measure the specific level of wastes in your blood and determine the level of function of your kidneys. Your doctor can figure out your kidney's filtration rate and identify your CKD stage based on this measurement.

There are five stages associated with CKD that correspond to how well your kidneys are functioning (see The Stages of Kidney Disease, page 5). During the early stages, people often do not experience any symptoms, and the disease can be very manageable. Kidney disease can even go undetected until it is quite advanced. Many symptoms do not begin to appear until the later stages, when toxins begin to build up in the body from damage to the kidneys. For example, itching, swelling, nausea, vomiting, or changes in urine patterns may be the result of the decreased filtration ability of these organs. That's why early diagnosis is so crucial and can result in very positive outcomes later on with regard to the disease's progression.

Although there is no cure for CKD, this disease is completely manageable. Making changes to your diet and lifestyle can help slow the progression of the disease and avoid symptoms that typically begin to emerge later on. These diet and lifestyle changes can even improve your overall health and help you manage associated conditions. As we will explore in the next few sections, there are associated diseases that may have led to CKD or perhaps were a contributing factor. When you begin making changes to your food and daily habits, you will also begin to notice improvement in these associated conditions, including hypertension and diabetes.

It is very possible to live a long, healthy, and happy life while managing this disease, and making the proper changes early on can slow the progression of any adverse symptoms for several years. I hope this book will shed this important light on you and your loved ones, so together we can make positive changes that delay the progression of CKD for a long time to come.

How Kidneys Work

The kidneys are a team of bean-shaped filters with a critical job—they regulate the stability of the entire body. Using different signals from the body, such as sodium content or blood-vessel pressure, the kidneys help regulate blood pressure and keep us well hydrated. For example, have you ever had a busy day and didn't get a chance to drink as much water as usual? Your mouth was parched, and you felt sluggish. Then, maybe you even noticed that your urine color was a bit too dark. That is the kidneys, keeping as much water in your body as possible and letting out all of the other things you don't need. When you are well hydrated, your urine is more diluted, because the kidneys realize that you don't need that much water to be held back, and they let it go through.

When the kidneys stop functioning properly, a series of problems can occur. Normal filtration of toxins slows down, and the buildup of these harmful chemicals can cause subsequent reactions in the body, such as rashes, nausea, or vomiting. As kidney function continues to decrease, the body's ability to remove water from the body and secrete hormones to control blood pressure is also affected, so symptoms like swelling of the feet or high blood pressure may occur. Over time, since the kidneys can stimulate the production of red blood cells from bone marrow, as well as create an active form of vitamin D, reduced kidney function can result in long-term health issues, like anemia or osteoporosis.

Our kidneys work hard, so it's important to protect them. In fact, they filter between 120 and 150 quarts of blood every day. This process produces 1 to 2 quarts of urine, which is made up of waste products and excess fluid.

Common Causes

Part of the management of kidney disease comes with understanding how you developed it. Preexisting conditions such as diabetes and hypertension are commonly associated with kidney disease and play a key role in decreasing the function of these organs. If you have these conditions, your dietary needs will be different, so it is important to consult with your doctor about what factors to consider as you begin adjusting your diet and lifestyle. In the next few sections, I'll help you understand the common causes of CKD and what to consider if you are juggling more than one condition.

Diabetes

Diabetes is a disease that alters your body's ability to either produce or use insulin. Insulin is a hormone released from the pancreas, which pulls sugar from the blood and sends it to the organs that require it for normal functioning. If you have diabetes, there is a good chance that you know all of this information in more detail, and you have been managing it with diet and medical treatment.

However, chronic or uncontrolled diabetes can be very damaging to the kidneys and play a major role in the development of CKD. In fact, diabetes is the leading cause of kidney disease. As mentioned, one of the kidney's jobs is to filter all the fluid in your body and let out the waste products along with excess water. Imagine this fluid hitting the filter of the kidney repeatedly, all day long. Luckily, our filtration system is typically strong enough to handle that pressure. However, when there are large molecules of sugar in our blood, this increases the pressure put on the filter, and eventually, it can break.

Relationships with your health care providers should be based on trust and respect, and the ability to rely on them for guidance and support.

If you have diabetes and are diagnosed with CKD, it is important to work with your doctor and a dietitian to create a twofold diet that (1) avoids the nutrients that should be limited with kidney disease and (2) controls your blood glucose levels. This book will provide specific recipes to help you get started.

High Blood Pressure/Hypertension

High blood pressure, also known as hypertension, can cause kidney damage and can be caused by kidney damage. Our blood vessels push all of our blood through the body—that blood puts pressure on the walls of our arteries. If the pressure is too high, it can begin to damage the walls of these vessels, especially smaller blood vessels like those found in the kidneys. Blood vessels that run through our kidneys exchange molecules during the filtration process, but damage to these walls can impede the work of the filtration system and cause damage to the kidneys, leading to CKD.

A primary function of the kidneys is to control blood pressure by producing certain hormones. If the kidneys become damaged, their ability to regulate these hormones decreases, and blood pressure can increase. If you are struggling with chronic hypertension or are looking to regulate your blood pressure due to CKD, diet and lifestyle management can help. Many key elements of a kidney-friendly diet also aid in managing hypertension, so it is important to consider this as you determine what kinds of positive changes you can make for your health.

THE STAGES OF KIDNEY DISEASE

For most individuals with kidney disease, progression of the disease is slow and occurs over a period of years. This is encouraging, because if CKD is caught early, interventions such as regular checkups, medicine, and lifestyle changes can greatly help slow its progression for a better quality of life.

The National Kidney Foundation (NKF) has created guidelines to help doctors identify the five levels of kidney disease. Each stage calls for different tests and treatments and is determined by the glomerular filtration rate (GFR). GFR is calculated using a person's age, race, gender, and serum creatinine (waste product of muscle breakdown). It is the most effective way to measure the level at which your kidneys are functioning.

This book is designed for individuals with CKD stages 1 through 4, to help slow or avoid the progression to CKD stage 5. Stage 5 may be indicative of kidney failure and the need for dialysis treatment.

Treating CKD

Effectively managing CKD requires a combination of dietary changes, lifestyle modifications, and partnership with health care providers. You can increase the chance for positive outcomes by educating yourself about the disease and learning as much as you can about the personal choices you can make as a patient. Knowledge truly is power, so gather all that you can! With CKD, this is especially true when it comes to your diet.

Diet

The "CKD 1–4 diet" can be overwhelming at first, but like anything new, once you begin to put it into practice, it will become a natural part of your lifestyle that requires little thought. The basic guidelines of the CKD 1–4 diet are restriction of protein, sodium, potassium, phosphorus, and in some cases, fluids. Based on your blood-work results and other factors, your dietitian and/or health care provider can create an individualized diet prescription for you. The rest is up to you; in fact, how well you comply with these dietary restrictions has enormous influence over the rate of disease progression.

This book focuses on a wide variety of foods that can be included in the CKD 1–4 diet. It provides examples of daily meal plans that are easy and quick to prepare, corresponding shopping lists, and 100 practical recipes to suit everyone's tastes. We all have good and bad days, and diet slipups may happen. Remember, it's not about perfection but what you do most of the time that matters!

STAGES OF CKD

- **Stage 1** Slight kidney damage with normal or increased filtration (GFR > 90 mL/min)

- **Stage 2** Mild decrease in kidney function (GFR = 60–89 mL/min)

- **Stage 3** Moderate decrease in kidney function (GFR = 30–59 mL/min)

- **Stage 4** Severe decrease in kidney function (GFR = 15–29 mL/min)

- **Stage 5** Kidney failure/ End-stage CKD (GFR < 15 mL/min)

Lifestyle

Like diet, lifestyle choices play a big part in CKD 1–4 management. Engaging in regular exercise, adequate sleep, good weight management, stress reduction, and avoiding cigarettes and alcohol are all healthy lifestyle practices. They can help you manage or reduce your risk of chronic diseases associated with CKD, like diabetes, cardiovascular disease, and high blood pressure. Thoughtful lifestyle choices, especially when practiced consistently, can make a huge difference in how you feel, both physically and emotionally.

Your Health Care Team

Treatment and management of your CKD should involve your health care team, inclusive of renal doctors, nurses, social workers, and a dietitian. These people each offer specific expertise, and together they are a comprehensive professional support system to educate and guide you with your CKD. As experts in the renal field, health care professionals are your best source of

GETTING SUPPORT

Upon receiving the news of a CKD diagnosis, it is completely normal to experience a wide range of emotions: fear, anxiety, sadness, anger, denial, and others. It's also common to experience these emotions as you start learning more about CKD, its impact on your life, and what changes you need to implement to help manage it. It can be overwhelming and devastating, and can affect you both physically and emotionally. But we live in a progressive society with countless valuable resources. Health care providers, physicians, social workers, nurses, and dietitians, to name a few, are available to listen, educate,

and support you through this new diagnosis. Do not feel you need to deal with this by yourself. Discussing your feelings with family, friends, and other CKD patients may be hugely reassuring and beneficial. Be open and honest with your providers so they can help you or refer you to other resources for support. Support groups and credible Internet sites (see Resources, page 185) are wonderful outlets that can help you learn more about your condition and its treatment, gain perspective on your situation, and put you in touch with others who are in a similar situation and can relate.

information. Encourage them to work together to develop an individualized plan of care that works for you. In order for your health care team to help you best, be open and honest with how you are feeling and the lifestyle and diet choices you're making. They are there not to judge but to help you make good choices in managing your CKD.

FAQs

Q: *There are so many things I can't eat now—what* can *I eat?*

A: What you should eat and how much is determined by what stage of CKD you are in. Routine checkups and lab work will help determine your food restrictions. This book is a guide that focuses on kidney-supportive foods—and the list is a long one! However, a registered dietitian (RD) can also help you sort out what foods to avoid and, more importantly, what foods you can have. An RD can help you develop personalized diet parameters and create practical individualized meal plans and lists of foods to meet your dietary needs to supplement those discussed in this book. A good RD can answer your questions and empower you to make your own smart and satisfying food choices.

Is there a cure for CKD?

There is no cure for CKD. However, there are many ways to manage the disease and live a long, full, productive life. If you have CKD, it is very important to have regular checkups, take your medication as prescribed, and follow your CKD diet/meal plan to slow the progression of the disease. The one thing you have complete control over is the choice of what and how much you eat. Diet compliance is one of the most important components of your health, as it influences your future health and well-being.

What can cause CKD?

Over time, other chronic diseases, such as diabetes, hypertension, or heart disease, can cause CKD. It can also be genetic or linked to ethnicities such as Native American, Hispanic, African American, or Asian. Age is another factor; people over 60 years old are at a higher risk for CKD.

Can I exercise if I have CKD?

Absolutely! Exercising at least 30 minutes, five days a week, can help keep symptoms in check and control associated factors, such as diabetes and hypertension.

What is a glomerular filtration rate (GFR) and why do I keep seeing numbers associated with this term?

The GFR is used to measure how well your kidneys are functioning. This number is used along with the amount of creatinine in your blood to calculate what stage of CKD you may be in, so it is important to talk to your doctor about these tests.

How can I tell if my CKD is getting worse?

Many symptoms are not noticeable until the advanced stages of CKD. It is important to begin adopting a kidney-friendly diet and lifestyle before your condition worsens. Regular checkups are helpful and reassuring, as your provider can monitor your levels and answer your questions. If you notice symptoms such as swelling, constant fatigue, changes in appetite, foamy urine, or trouble with concentration, please contact your doctor.

If I have CKD, am I going to need dialysis?

CKD, especially if caught early, can be controlled, and advanced stages can be delayed with proper nutrition and lifestyle changes. In fact, only about 1 out of 50 people who are diagnosed with CKD progress to kidney failure and the need for dialysis. CKD does result in a higher risk for other complications, such as heart disease or stroke; this is one more good reason to work with your doctor and dietitian to manage your diet and medications and prevent any further damage.

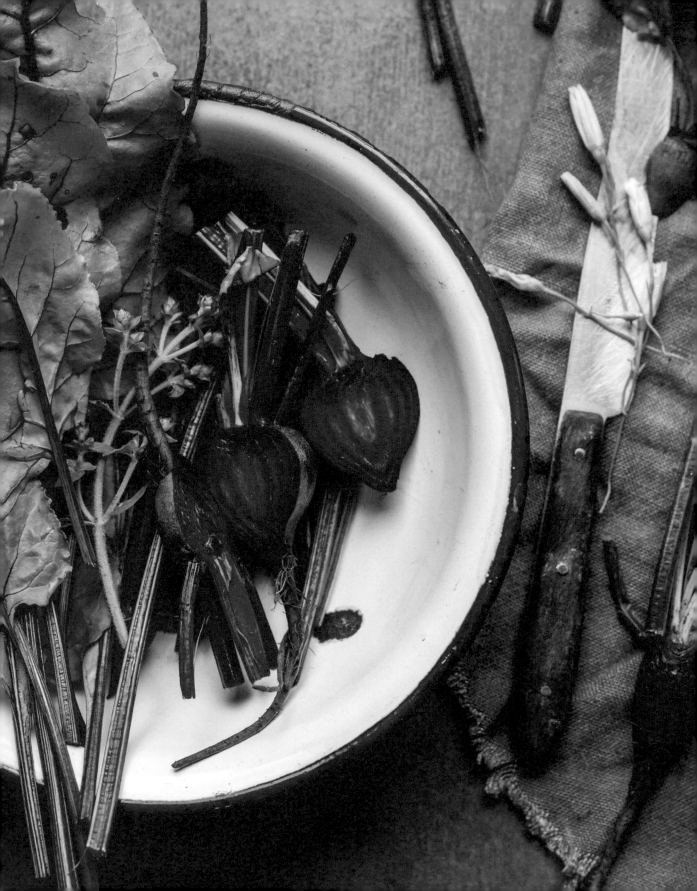

CHAPTER TWO

Slowing Kidney Disease in 5 Steps

In this chapter, we'll explore five steps to adopting a renal diet. I will share important information for you to know, and will arm you with specific action steps to adopt a healthy diet and lifestyle. Keep an open mind, and we will take this one step at a time, together! A positive attitude is most important, and how you embrace the following steps will greatly determine how well you manage your kidney disease. As an experienced professional in this field, I promise to give you all the tools you need to succeed, and with a little determination from your end and some good old-fashioned willpower, you will be in charge of your health and destiny in no time.

Step 1: Make a Commitment

You've been diagnosed with kidney disease, and there are probably a million things running through your mind. No doubt you're feeling a little overwhelmed. Take a deep breath, and another one. I can tell you that it's going to be okay, because you are in charge. Sure, like any change in life, new habits take time to develop. So take it one day at a time. Begin by preparing yourself mentally by meditating on the fact that your kidney disease *can* be controlled by how you manage your diet and lifestyle. Make a promise to yourself that you will try your best each and every day to change your dietary habits and lifestyle. Your personal commitment to yourself and your desire and motivation to follow through will have everything to do with how well you can manage your kidney disease. Remember, the earlier your kidney disease is detected, the sooner it can be treated. The goals of your treatment are twofold: to slow kidney disease and to prevent it from getting worse. That's one unique thing about kidney disease: It will allow you to take control of managing it.

Step 2: Understand Your Nutrient Needs

There is no one eating plan that is right for everyone with kidney disease. What you can or cannot eat will change over time, depending on your kidney function and other factors, like having diabetes, for example. By working closely with your health care providers and continuing to educate yourself, you can master the art of making healthy food choices to fit your needs and will be able to personally manage your disease with tremendous success.

The following are some basic dietary guidelines useful to all individuals with chronic kidney disease (CKD).

Protein

Protein can be found in foods from both animals and plants. Protein is a necessary macronutrient for a healthy body; however, for CKD patients, too much is not a good thing. As kidney function declines, the body loses the ability to remove waste produced by the breakdown of protein, so it starts to build up in the blood. The right amount of protein intake for you is dependent on your stage of kidney disease, nutritional status (such as albumin level and appetite), body size, and other factors. A registered dietitian can help you calculate your daily protein limits. As a guide, I've provided a list of lean sources of high-quality protein to choose from, with suggested serving sizes, in the table "High-Protein Foods."

If you have kidney disease and smoke, your risk increases for end-stage renal disease. According to the Centers for Disease Control and Prevention, smoking harms nearly every organ of the body. Stopping may be the most important preventive measure you can take. Ask your doctor about nicotine-replacement options.

High-Protein Foods

SEAFOOD, MEAT, AND POULTRY*	VEGETABLES, LEGUMES, AND NUTS**	BREADS, CEREALS, AND GRAINS***	DAIRY, EGGS, AND SOY****
• Beef	• Almonds, whole, 7 or 8	• Bagel, ½	• Cheese (hard cheeses such as Cheddar, mozzarella, Swiss, Gouda, Colby), 1 ounce
• Chicken	• Beans, canned	• Bread, 1 slice	
• Clams, 5 small or 2 large	• Beans, green and wax	• Biscuit or roll, 1	• Cream (coffee cream, half-and-half)
• Fish	• Broccoli	• Bun (hamburger or roll), ½	
• Lamb	• Cabbage, green and red	• Cereals, cold (Cheerios, Corn Flakes, puffed rice), 1 cup	• Cream soups
• Shrimp or scallops, 4	• Carrots	• Cereals, hot (oatmeal, grits, rice, Cream of Wheat/farina), ½ cup	• Cottage cheese, ¼ cup
• Pork	• Cauliflower		• Edamame
• Tuna or salmon, ⅛ cup or 1 ounce	• Celery	• Cornbread, homemade, 1 (2-inch) cube	• Eggs, 1 medium; egg whites; or egg substitute, ¼ cup
	• Coleslaw	• Crackers (unsalted or graham crackers), 10	
• Turkey	• Cucumbers	• Muffin, homemade, 1	• Ice cream
	• Eggplant	• Pancakes or waffles, homemade, 1 (4-inch diameter)	• Milk, whole, 2%, 1%, fat-free (skim), soy milk
	• Escarole		
	• Greens, mustard, turnip	• Pasta or rice, cooked ½ cup	• Pudding and custard
	• Lentils, ⅛ cup	• Pita bread pocket, ½	• Tofu, ¼ cup
	• Lettuce	• Popcorn (unsalted), 2 cups	• Yogurt, plain
	• Peanut butter or nut butters, 2 tablespoons	• Tortilla, 1	
	• Peas, green, canned		

*One serving = 1 ounce, providing about 7 grams of protein unless otherwise noted.
**One serving = ½ cup, providing about 2 grams of protein unless otherwise noted.
***One serving = varies by food, providing about 2 to 3 grams of protein.
****One serving = ½ cup, providing about 4 to 6 grams of protein unless otherwise noted.

Fats

In a time of restriction, it may feel like good news to know that healthy fat in moderation is an important macronutrient to include on a daily basis. The consumption of healthy fats ensures you are getting essential fatty acids, which help the body in numerous ways. Monounsaturated and polyunsaturated fats are both unsaturated fats; they're considered the healthiest of the fats due to their potential cardiovascular health benefits (including lowering total cholesterol, increasing HDL cholesterol, and decreasing LDL cholesterol). The right kinds of fats may also decrease inflammation in the body and protect your kidneys from further damage. Include small amounts of the following healthy fats in your diet.

MONOUNSATURATED FATS
(healthy fats, liquid at room temperature)

- Avocados
- Olive oil
- Peanut oil
- Sesame oil
- Some safflower oil (high in oleic acid)

POLYUNSATURATED FATS

- Corn oil
- Fish, such as salmon, mackerel, herring, albacore tuna, and trout
- Flaxseed or flax oil
- Some safflower oil (high in linoleic acid)
- Soybean oil
- Sunflower seeds
- Walnuts

Carbohydrates

Carbohydrates are an important macronutrient needed by the body. They are the body's major source of fuel to provide energy. They also offer a wide range of vitamins, minerals, and fiber that help protect your body. Here are some renal-friendly sources of high-fiber carbohydrates to include in your diet on a daily basis, with suggested serving sizes, in the table "High-Fiber Foods."

High-Fiber Foods*

FRUITS (1–4g fiber)	VEGETABLES (1–4g fiber)	BREADS AND GRAINS (1–8.5g fiber)
• Apple, raw with skin, 2.5 grams	• Asparagus, 1.4 grams	• Air-popped popcorn, 1 cup, 1.2 grams
• Applesauce, 3 grams	• Beans, green/yellow, 3.4 grams	• Barley, pearled, cooked, 6 grams
• Apricot, halves, 1.5 grams	• Broccoli, 1.1 grams	• Bread, white, 2 slices, 1.6 grams
• Blackberries, 4 grams	• Cabbage, raw, 1.1 grams	• Buckwheat, cooked, 8.5 grams
• Blueberries, 1.8 grams	• Carrots, 1.8 grams	
• Cherries, 1 cup, 3 grams	• Cauliflower, cooked, 1 gram	• Bulgur, cooked, 4.1 grams
• Cranberries, raw, 2.5 grams	• Corn, cooked, 1.8 grams	• Corn grits, yellow, cooked, 1 cup, 1 gram
• Grapes, red or green, 1 cup, 1.5 grams	• Peas, frozen, cooked, 4 grams	• Corn Flakes, 1 cup, 1 gram
• Peach, 1 large, 2.6 grams	• Zucchini, cooked, 1 cup, 1.8 grams	• Flaxseed, whole, 1 tablespoon, 2.8 grams
• Pear, raw with skin, 3 grams		• Grape-Nuts Flakes, ¾ cup, 3 grams
• Pineapple, 1 cup, 2.3 grams		• Polenta, cooked, 1.5 grams
• Raspberries, 4 grams		• Rice, brown, cooked, 1.7 grams
• Strawberries, sliced, 1.7 grams		• Rice, long-grain white, cooked, 1 gram
• Tangerine, 1.8 grams		

*One serving = ½ cup unless otherwise noted.

Sodium

Too much sodium can make you thirsty, which can lead to swelling and increased blood pressure. High blood pressure can cause more damage to unhealthy kidneys. Eating less sodium helps lower blood pressure and may slow down CKD. The recommendation is for people with CKD to limit sodium intake to 2,000 milligrams per day. For best success in this area, remember "fresh is best." Sodium is found abundantly in any food that has been processed, salted, cured, or pickled. Canned, frozen convenience, and fast foods tend to be very high in sodium. Conversely, the less processed a food is, the less sodium is added. If the "fresh is best" concept is a lifestyle change for you, be assured, this book has lots of delectable recipes that eliminate the salt and allow for discovery of other creative ways to season your food.

Did you know that your attitude influences how you feel? Make it a point to surround yourself with positive and supportive people and pursue activities that make you happy. A sunny outlook is proven to result in better health!

One of the best things that you can do to stay healthy is to limit how much sodium you eat. To do so, here are some "sodium swaps" you can try.

Sodium in Common Foods

TYPE OF FOOD	CHOOSE	AVOID/LIMIT
VEGETABLES	Fresh, frozen, or unsalted canned vegetables	Canned tomato juice or sauce, canned vegetables, vegetable juice, sauerkraut, pickled vegetables, olives
FRUIT	Fresh, frozen, or canned fruit Fruit juices	
BREADS/ CEREALS/ STARCHES	Bread, rolls, pitas, tortillas, unsalted crackers Shredded or puffed wheat or rice Plain rice, pasta, noodles	Instant hot cereals, quick breads made with baking powder or baking soda (biscuit, pancake, waffle, muffin mixes), salted crackers or snack items Rice or pasta box mixes with seasoning packets (Rice-A-Roni/macaroni and cheese)
DAIRY	Milk, all types (½ cup) Yogurt Low-sodium cheese	Buttermilk, cottage cheese, processed cheese spread
MEATS/ PROTEIN	Fresh eggs, fish, poultry, pork, red meat Low-sodium deli meats	Lunch meat, ham, bacon, sausage, kielbasa, salt pork, corned beef, hot dogs, Spam
SNACK FOODS	Air-popped popcorn, no-salt pretzels or tortilla or corn chips, rice cakes, unsalted nuts	Potato chips, any salted snack food, salted nuts or seeds
HERBS, SPICES, SEASONINGS	Fresh and dried herbs and spices (any except those listed in the "Avoid" list), lemon juice, salt-free seasoning blends, vinegar	Table salt, seasoning salt, garlic salt, onion salt, celery salt, lemon pepper, Lite Salt, meat tenderizer, bouillon cubes, flavor enhancers
OTHER	Homemade or low-sodium soups, canned food without salt Homemade low- or no-sodium sauces, marinades, salad dressings Homemade casseroles without added salt, made with fresh or frozen vegetables, fresh meat, rice, pasta, unsalted canned vegetables	Barbecue sauce, ketchup, steak sauce, soy sauce, teriyaki sauce, oyster sauce Frozen dinners, frozen convenience foods (chicken nuggets, frozen pizzas, prepared meatballs, lasagnas, etc.) Canned ravioli/pastas Fast foods

Potassium

Potassium is found in many foods and beverages, and it plays an important role in regulating the heartbeat and keeping muscles functioning well. However, people with unhealthy kidneys often need to limit certain foods that can increase the potassium in the blood to a dangerous level. A potassium-restricted diet is typically about 2,000 milligrams per day. Your physician or dietitian can advise you as to the right potassium intake for you, based on blood work results and your individual health needs.

To reduce potassium buildup, you'll need to learn which foods are high in potassium and which are low, so you know which to be careful with. Refer to the following "Potassium in Common Foods" table to learn which foods are high and low in potassium so you can make safe, low-potassium food choices.

Potassium in Common Foods*

LOW POTASSIUM (Less than 150 mg/serving)	MEDIUM POTASSIUM (151–250 mg/serving)	HIGH POTASSIUM (More than 251 mg/serving)
• Alfalfa seeds, sprouted, raw	• Apple, without skin, 1 large	• Apricot, 1 cup
• Apple juice	• Apricot, halves, 1 medium	• Artichoke, 1 medium
• Applesauce, sweetened	• Apricots, in heavy syrup, drained	• Avocado
• Bagel, 1 plain (4-inch diameter)	• Asparagus, boiled, 5 spears	• Bamboo shoots, cooked
• Beans, green, frozen	• Beans, green, boiled, 1 cup	• Banana, 1 small
• Blueberries	• Blackberries, 1 cup	• Beans, black, mature, boiled
• Cabbage, shredded, boiled	• Broccoli, frozen, 1 cup	• Beans, dried
• Carrot, baby raw, 1 medium	• Brussels sprouts, boiled	• Beans, lima, large, mature, boiled, ⅓ cup
• Cherries, sour canned, in syrup	• Carrots, sliced, 1 cup	• Beans, pinto, mature, boiled
• Coffee, 1 cup	• Cereal, All-Bran	• Beans, refried, canned
• Cranberries, dried	• Cherries, 10 sweet	• Beets, cooked
• Cranberry juice	• Chickpeas, dried, boiled	• Cabbage, Chinese, cooked
• Cranberry sauce, canned	• Collards, chopped, frozen	• Cantaloupe, cubed, 1 cup
	• Corn, yellow, boiled, 1 ear	• Chard, Swiss, boiled, ⅓ cup

*One serving = ½ cup unless otherwise noted. ▶

Potassium in Common Foods*

LOW POTASSIUM (Less than 150 mg/serving)	MEDIUM POTASSIUM (151–250 mg/serving)	HIGH POTASSIUM (More than 251 mg/serving)
• Eggplant, boiled	• Date, dried, 1 date	• Chocolate
• Fig, raw, 1 medium	• Elderberries	• Dates, Medjool
• Ginger ale, 12 ounces	• Grapefruit, ½ medium	• Fruits, dried
• Grapes	• Grapefruit juice	• Mango, pieces, 1 cup
• Lemon, 1 medium	• Grape juice, 1 cup	• Milk, 1%, 1 cup
• Lime, 1 medium	• Honeydew melon, pieces	• Milk, soy, 1 cup
• Mustard greens, frozen	• Kiwifruit, 1 medium	• Milk, whole, 1 cup
• Oatmeal, regular	• Leeks, 1 raw	• Molasses, 1 tablespoon
• Okra, cooked	• Mustard greens, cooked, ¾ cup	• Mushrooms, cooked, 1 cup
• Onions, raw, diced	• Onion, chopped, boiled	• Nectarine, 1 medium
• Parsley, raw, 10 sprigs	• Orange, 1 medium	• Nuts, mixed, 2 ounces
• Peaches, canned, in syrup, drained	• Peach, 1 small	• Orange juice, fresh
• Pears, canned, in syrup, drained	• Pear, 1 medium	• Papaya, 1 small
• Peppers, sweet, cooked	• Peppers, hot chile	• Plantain, sliced, cooked
• Pineapple, pieces	• Peppers, sweet, raw	• Pomegranate, 1 small
• Plum, 1 medium	• Pineapple, canned	• Pomegranate juice
• Popcorn, buttered	• Pineapple juice	• Potatoes, white, baked, 1 medium
• Prunes, dried, 1 prune	• Prickly pear, 1 medium	• Raisins, seedless, 1.5-ounce box
• Radicchio, raw, shredded	• Prunes, canned, 5 prunes	• Sapodilla, 1 medium
• Raspberries	• Radishes, raw, sliced, 1 cup	• Sauerkraut, undrained, 1 cup
• Rhubarb, cooked with sugar	• Raspberries, frozen, sweetened, 1 cup	• Spinach, cooked
• Rice, white, enriched, 1 cup cooked	• Scallions, chopped, raw, 1 cup	• Succotash, boiled
• Spaghetti, enriched, cooked	• Squash, summer	• Sweet potatoes, boiled
• Spinach, raw, chopped	• Strawberries, whole, 1 cup	• Tomato, 1 medium
• Tea, black, 8 ounces	• Tangerine, 1 large	• Tomato paste, canned, ¼ cup
• Turnips, white, cubed	• Tortillas, corn, 4 (6-inch diameter)	• Tomato sauce, canned, ¼ cup
• Water chestnuts, canned	• Turnip greens, chopped	• Water chestnuts, raw
• Watermelon, pieces		

*One serving = ½ cup unless otherwise noted.

Phosphorus

Healthy kidneys help the body regulate phosphorus. However, with CKD, your kidneys are unable to remove excess phosphorus or excrete it. The end result is high phosphorus levels in the blood—this pulls calcium from the bones, which can lead to weak, brittle bones. Elevated levels of phosphorus and calcium in the blood can also lead to dangerous mineral deposits in the body's soft tissues, an ailment called calciphylaxis. Phosphorus is found both naturally in animal and plant proteins, and more abundantly in highly processed foods. You can maintain safe levels of phosphorus in your body by making smart low-phosphorus food choices. The rule of thumb to prevent consuming unwanted hidden phosphorus circles back to the concept "fresh is best"; that is, avoid processed foods. Daily phosphorus intake for individuals with CKD should be 800 to 1,000 milligrams. Please refer to the following "Phosphorus in Common Foods" table to help you make wise low-phosphorus food choices.

Phosphorus in Common Foods[*]

LOW PHOSPHORUS (Less than 150 mg/serving)	MEDIUM PHOSPHORUS (151-250 mg/serving)	HIGH PHOSPHORUS (More than 251 mg/serving)
• Apple	• Beans, black, 1 cup	• Peanuts, oil roasted, 2 ounces
• Bagel, 1 plain (4-inch diameter)	• Beans, fava, 1 cup	• Almonds, oil/dry roasted, 2 ounces
• Barley, pearled, cooked	• Beans, kidney, 1 cup	• Baked beans, 1 cup
• Beans, green	• Beans, pinto, 1 cup	• Beans, small white, mature, boiled, 1 cup
• Bread, pita, 1 (6.5-inch diameter)	• Beef, bottom round, 3 ounces	• Beef, liver, cooked, 3 ounces
• Bread, pumpernickel, 2 slices	• Beef, chuck roast, 3 ounces	• Beefalo, 3 ounces
• Bread, white, 2 slices	• Beef, eye round, 3 ounces	• Buttermilk, 1 cup
• Butter, 1 tablespoon	• Beef, ground, 70% lean, 3 ounces	• Calamari, fried, 3 ounces
	• Beef, ground, 95% lean, 3 ounces	

[*]One serving = ½ cup unless otherwise noted. ▶

Phosphorus in Common Foods[*]

LOW PHOSPHORUS (Less than 150 mg/serving)	MEDIUM PHOSPHORUS (151–250 mg/serving)	HIGH PHOSPHORUS (More than 251 mg/serving)
• Cabbage	• Beef, sirloin steak, 3 ounces	• Cashews, dry roasted, 2 ounces
• Cauliflower	• Black-eyed peas, 1 cup	• Cereal, bran, 100%
• Cereal, crispy rice, 1 cup	• Bread, whole-wheat, 2 slices	• Cereal, wheat-germ, ¼ cup
• Cheese, Brie, 1 ounce	• Catfish, breaded/fried, 3 ounces	• Cheese, goat, 2 ounces
• Cheese, feta, 1 ounce	• Cheese, blue, 2 ounces	• Cheese, Parmesan, 2 ounces
• Cocoa, unsweetened, 2 tablespoons	• Cheese, Cheddar, 1 ounce	• Cheese, ricotta, part skim
• Cookies, shortbread, 4	• Cheese, mozzarella, 1 ounce	• Cheese, Romano, 2 ounces
• Cornflakes, 1 cup	• Cheese, provolone, 2 ounces	• Chia seeds, 1 ounce
• Cottage cheese, nonfat	• Cheese, Swiss, 1 ounce	• Chicken, liver, cooked, 3 ounces
• Couscous, cooked	• Chicken, breast, 3 ounces	• Clam chowder, New England
• Cream cheese, 1 ounce	• Chicken, dark meat, 3 ounces	• Clams, cooked with moist heat, 3 ounces
• Cucumber	• Chickpeas, 1 cup	• Corn bread, 1 piece
• Duck, with skin, 3 ounces	• Chocolate, plain, 2 ounces	• Crab, Alaska king, cooked with moist heat, 3 ounces
• Egg white, 1 large	• Cod, Pacific, 3 ounces	• Custard, flan, 1 cup
• Egg yolk, 1 large	• Cottage cheese, 1% fat	• Flounder, 3 ounces
• Eggplant	• Cottage cheese, 2% fat	• Halibut, Atlantic/Pacific, 3 ounces
• English muffin, 1 plain	• Crab, blue, cooked with moist heat, 3 ounces	• Lentils, mature, boiled, 1 cup
• Figs	• Crab, Dungeness, cooked with moist heat, 3 ounces	• Milk, 1%, 1 cup
• Gelatin, water base	• Lamb, kebabs, domestic, 3 ounces	• Milk, chocolate, 1 cup
• Ginger ale, 1 can	• Lamb, leg roast, domestic, 3 ounces	• Milk, evaporated, nonfat
• Grapefruit	• Lamb, New Zealand, 3 ounces	• Milk, nonfat, 1 cup
• Grapes	• Lobster, cooked with moist heat, 3 ounces	• Milk, whole, 1 cup
• Grouper		• Mussels, blue, cooked with moist heat, 3 ounces
• Hominy grits		• Nuts, Brazil, 2 ounces
• Ice cream, 10% fat, vanilla		• Nuts, pine, 2 ounces
• Lettuce		
• Milk, soy, 1 cup		
• Oatmeal, cooked, 1 packet		

[*]One serving = ½ cup unless otherwise noted.

Phosphorus in Common Foods[*]

LOW PHOSPHORUS (Less than 150 mg/serving)	MEDIUM PHOSPHORUS (151–250 mg/serving)	HIGH PHOSPHORUS (More than 251 mg/serving)
• Onions	• Macadamia nuts, 3 ounces	• Oysters, Eastern, cooked with moist heat, 3 ounces
• Oysters, canned, 3 ounces	• Milk, canned, sweetened, condensed, ¼ cup	• Peanuts, boiled, 1 cup
• Oysters, raw, Pacific, 3 ounces	• Mushrooms, cooked, 1 cup	• Peanuts, dry roasted, 3 ounces
• Pasta, 1 cup	• Mussels, raw, blue, 3 ounces	• Peanuts, oil roasted, 2 ounces
• Peas, split, mature, boiled	• Peanut butter, 2 tablespoons	• Pecans, oil/dry roasted, 3 ounces
• Plums	• Pork, boneless loin chop, 3 ounces	• Salmon, canned, pink/red, 3 ounces
• Popcorn, air-popped, 1 cup	• Pork, leg roast, 3 ounces	• Sardines, canned in oil, 3 ounces
• Pork, spare ribs, 3 ounces	• Raisin Bran, 1 cup	• Scallops, breaded/fried, 3 ounces
• Radishes	• Raisins, seedless, 1 cup	• Sole, 3 ounces
• Rice cakes, 1 cake	• Rice, brown, cooked, 1 cup	• Soybeans, mature, boiled
• Rice, white, enriched, cooked	• Shredded Wheat, 1 cup	• Sunflower seeds, 1 ounce
• Sherbet	• Shrimp, breaded/fried, 3 ounces	• Swordfish, 3 ounces
• Shrimp, cooked with moist heat, 3 ounces	• Snapper, 3 ounces	• Tofu, raw, firm
• Sour cream	• Spinach, raw	• Tuna, light, canned in oil, 3 ounces
• Tofu, soft	• Tortilla, 2 corn or flour (6-inch diameter)	• Tuna, white, canned in oil, 3 ounces
• Wheat flour, white, 1 cup	• Turkey, breast, 3 ounces	• Veal, cubed, stewed, 3 ounces
	• Turkey, dark meat, 3 ounces	• Walnuts, English, 2 ounces
	• Veal, rib roast, 3 ounces	• Wheat flour, whole-grain, 1 cup
	• Wheat flakes, 1 cup	• Yogurt, low-fat
		• Yogurt, skim

[*]One serving = ½ cup unless otherwise noted.

Vitamins and Supplements

Rather than just relying on supplements, following a balanced diet is the preferred way to get the recommended amount of daily vitamins. However, due to the restrictive nature of the CKD diet, it can be challenging to get all the necessary vitamins and nutrients you need on a daily basis. People with CKD have greater requirements for some water-soluble vitamins. Special renal vitamin supplements are also recommended to provide the necessary extra water-soluble vitamins. Renal vitamins contain vitamins B_1, B_2, B_6, and B_{12}, as well as folic acid, niacin, pantothenic acid, biotin, and a small dose of vitamin C.

One of the kidneys' functions is to convert inactive vitamin D to active vitamin D so the body is able to use it. With CKD, the kidneys lose this ability. Your doctor may check your calcium, phosphorus, and PTH (parathyroid hormone) levels to determine if you need supplementation of active vitamin D, which is available by prescription only.

If your doctor has not prescribed a vitamin supplement, don't hesitate to ask if you could benefit from taking one. For the benefit of your health, use only vitamin supplements approved by your kidney doctor or dietitian.

RECAP: KIDNEY DISEASE AND YOUR DIET

- Limit your daily protein intake to the amount calculated by your health care team. Choose lean, high-value protein sources.

- Use heart-healthy fats (mono- and polyunsaturated) in moderation.

- Choose high-fiber carbohydrates.

- Limit sodium intake to 2,000 milligrams per day. Avoid highly processed foods that contain a lot of sodium. Try cooking with fresh, whole ingredients to create low-sodium meals.

- Limit potassium intake to 2,000 milligrams per day.

- Limit phosphorus to 800 to 1,000 milligrams per day.

- Ask your physician about the benefits of a daily renal vitamin.

- Fluid intake restrictions may not be necessary for CKD 1–4. Discuss your individual daily fluid needs with your health care team.

Fluids

One of the main functions of the kidneys is to regulate fluid balance in the body. For most individuals with CKD, fluid restriction isn't necessary as long as urine output is normal. As CKD progresses, there is a decline in urine output and an increase in fluid retention. When this occurs, fluid restrictions are necessary. Always pay close attention to the volume of your urine output, and tell your health care team if you find it is declining. They can best inform you on how much fluid to limit yourself to on a daily basis in order to maintain healthy fluid levels and help prevent fluid overload and medical complications associated with excess fluid buildup (such as edema, high blood pressure, congestive heart failure, and pulmonary edema).

WORKSHEET: My Renal Diet

Working closely with your health care team is important to establish health-supportive personal dietary needs and goals. Many factors are considered when calculating an individual's dietary needs: stage of renal disease, concurrent medical issues, lab results, and other variables. By learning as much as you can about your specific daily dietary needs, you can make smart, healthy food choices on your own that will reward you with good health. Use the following chart to log your dietary needs. From there, you can navigate this book and utilize all of its resources, from lists of foods to eat and not to eat, to shopping lists, daily meal plans, kidney-friendly recipes, and other helpful tools that will help you meet your personal daily nutrition needs and provide reassurance that you're doing the best for your body. To calculate your nutrient needs, talk with your physician and/or dietitian. The number varies person to person depending on your height, weight, and laboratory values.

My Renal Diet

NUTRIENT	MY NEEDS
PROTEIN	
FATS	
SODIUM	
POTASSIUM	
PHOSPHORUS	
CARBOHYDRATES	
VITAMINS	

Step 3: Know Your Daily Caloric Requirements

Daily caloric requirements vary from person to person, whether they have CKD or not. With CKD, eating enough calories and choosing the right foods can benefit your body more than ever before. Calories provide energy and help us function on a daily basis. They can also help prevent infection, avoid muscle-mass loss, maintain a healthy weight, and slow down the progression of kidney disease. However, if your caloric intake is too high, you will likely gain weight, which can put an additional burden on your kidneys. It is very important to get just the right number of calories. Caloric requirements for anyone with CKD are 30 to 35 calories per kilogram of body weight. For example, if you weigh 150 pounds, you need about 2,000 calories per day for optimal performance.

Step 4: Read Nutrition Labels

The renal diet takes some time to learn and put into practice. Luckily, all packaged food products come with a nutrition facts label and ingredients list. Reading these labels can be a real eye-opener! Let's explore what to look for and how to decipher the information on the label, so you can make educated food choices to meet your personal nutrition needs. Reading labels can prove an essential tool for selecting renal-appropriate foods—a good habit to develop in general.

CALORIE CALCULATOR

Many factors come into play when calculating how many calories you need on a daily basis. Your height, weight, age, gender, and the level of your physical activity are all considerations. That said, it is very easy to calculate your daily caloric needs. You can do it online with a tool created by the National Institute of Diabetes and Digestive and Kidney Diseases, and it takes only a few seconds. Visit www.supertracker .usda.gov/bwp/index.html for more information.

The most important ingredients that individuals with CKD need to look for on the food labels are fat, sodium, phosphorus, and potassium. By law, food manufacturers are required to list the fat and sodium content of a food. However, they are not required to list phosphorus or potassium content. Therefore, it's important to obtain this information in other ways, such as from the lists in this book or the Internet.

(A) *Serving size:* This information is provided in familiar units that consumers use (1 cup, 15 cookies, etc.).

(B) *Servings per container:* This indicates how many servings of food are in the container. Note: All nutrient values listed are for *one* serving of food.

(C) *Calories:* This is the number of calories in *one* serving of food.

(D) *Total fat:* This is the total content of all fats—unhealthy and healthy—in *one* serving of food. Note: By law, food manufacturers are required to list only the unhealthy fat content in a food (saturated and trans fats), due to their role in the development of cardiovascular disease.

Nutrition Facts

(A) Serving Size 1 cup (110g)
Servings Per Container About 6 **(B)**

Amount Per Serving

(C) Calories 250   Calories from Fat 30

	% Daily Value*
Total Fat 7g **(D)**	**11%**
Saturated Fat 3g	**16%**
Trans Fat 0g	
Cholesterol 4mg	**2%**
(E) Sodium 300mg	**13%**
Total Carbohydrate 30g	**10%**
Dietary Fiber 3g	**14%**
Sugars 2g	
Protein 5g	

Vitamin A	7%
Vitamin C	15%
Calcium	20%
Iron	32%

* Percent Daily Values are based on a 2,000 calorie diet. Your daily value may be higher or lower depending on your calorie needs.

	Calories:	2,000	2,500
Total Fat	Less than	55g	75g
Saturated Fat	Less than	10g	12g
Cholesterol	Less than	1,500mg	1,700mg
Total Carbohydrate		250mg	300mg
Dietary Fiber		22mg	31mg

- Look for foods that have 2 grams or less of saturated or trans saturated fats per serving.
- Healthy fats—monounsaturated and polyunsaturated fats (which are not required to be listed but still may be in the food item)—should be consumed in moderation.
- Choose foods that have less than 3 grams of total fat per serving, which is considered low-fat.
- Some nutrient claims on labels can also be useful in selecting heart-healthy food items. Look for claims like "saturated fat-free," "sodium-free," "low saturated fat," and "no trans fat."

(E) **Sodium:** As mentioned, the recommended daily intake of sodium is limited to about 2,000 milligrams. The Food and Drug Administration mandates that milligrams of sodium per serving must be listed for all food items. This takes the guesswork out of determining if that food item is renal-friendly or not.

Low-sodium foods: Look for those containing less than 140 milligrams per serving.

High-sodium foods: Avoid foods containing more than 500 milligrams per serving.

Nutrient claims on labels can also help guide your food selections. Look for "very low sodium," "low sodium," and "reduced salt." Foods must meet certain requirements to use these claims.

Phosphorus: Most CKD patients are limited to between 800 and 1,000 milligrams of phosphorus per day (your specific needs can be determined by your health care team). Phosphorus content is not required by law to be listed on the nutrient facts label, but here's a trick to get that information from the ingredients list. To determine if a food product has had phosphorus added, look for any ingredient that contains the four letters "phos." Phosphorus is naturally occurring in animal and plant protein sources, so foods that have added phosphorus should be avoided completely. If phosphorus additives are on the ingredient list, do yourself a favor and put that food product back on the shelf.

Phosphorus additives include the following:

- **Phos**phoric acid
- Sodium poly**phos**phate
- Pyro**phos**phate
- Sodium tripoly**phos**phate
- Poly**phos**phate
- Tricalcium **phos**phate
- Hexameta**phos**phate

- Trisodium **phos**phate
- Dicalcium **phos**phate
- Sodium **phos**phate
- Monocalcium **phos**phate
- Tetrasodium **phos**phate
- Aluminum **phos**phate

Potassium: Most CKD patients are limited to about 2,000 milligrams of potassium per day (your specific needs can be determined by your health care team). Potassium is another nutrient that is not required by law to be listed on the nutrient facts label, but you can get some helpful information by reading the ingredients list. Potassium is naturally occurring in many fruits, vegetables, and dairy products, but it can also be added for flavor and as a preservative to many processed foods.

Want to learn more about the foods you eat (or want to eat)? The Environmental Working Group rates thousands of food products and provides nutritional information as well. Visit EWD.org/foodscores.

Steer clear of food items that have any potassium additives, such as the following:

- Potassium acetates
- Potassium alginate
- Potassium alum
- Potassium bisulfite
- Potassium bromate
- Potassium carbonate
- Potassium caseinate

- Potassium chloride
- Potassium citrates
- Potassium gluconate
- Potassium hydroxide
- Potassium nitrate
- Potassium phosphates

Step 5: Practice Portion Control

Portion control is very important when you have kidney disease, but that doesn't mean you have to go hungry. Whatever stage of CKD you're in, eating in moderation is important to preserving kidney health, but the idea is not to feel deprived; rather, you can enjoy a variety of kidney-friendly foods without overeating. When you watch what you eat, and cut back on certain foods that can be harmful to your health, you are practicing portion control. Making a habit of eating in moderation and limiting certain foods on a kidney diet is yours to achieve—all it takes is a little time, some resolve, and an informed game plan.

Choosing the right foods on a renal diet is crucial to your kidneys; they're counting on you to provide the right amount of nutrients to help them function at their best, including protein, carbohydrates, fats, vitamins, and minerals. Too much of any nutrient can be harmful to your body and require your kidneys to work extra hard to filter out the toxins.

One way to get used to portion control and choosing the right foods is by practicing the strategy of balancing your plate. Visualize your plate made up of ½ vegetables, ¼ protein, and ¼ carbohydrates, as pictured below.

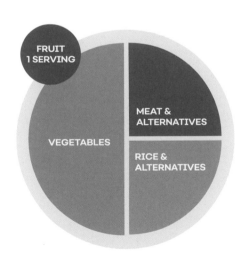

I've packed a lot of information in these first two chapters, and it will take some time to remember it all. That's okay; just take it one day at a time and stay committed to learning and achieving. By keeping this book on hand, you can return to these early chapters as often as necessary. Before long, you'll be an expert on your body, knowing what it needs to thrive and sustain good kidney health.

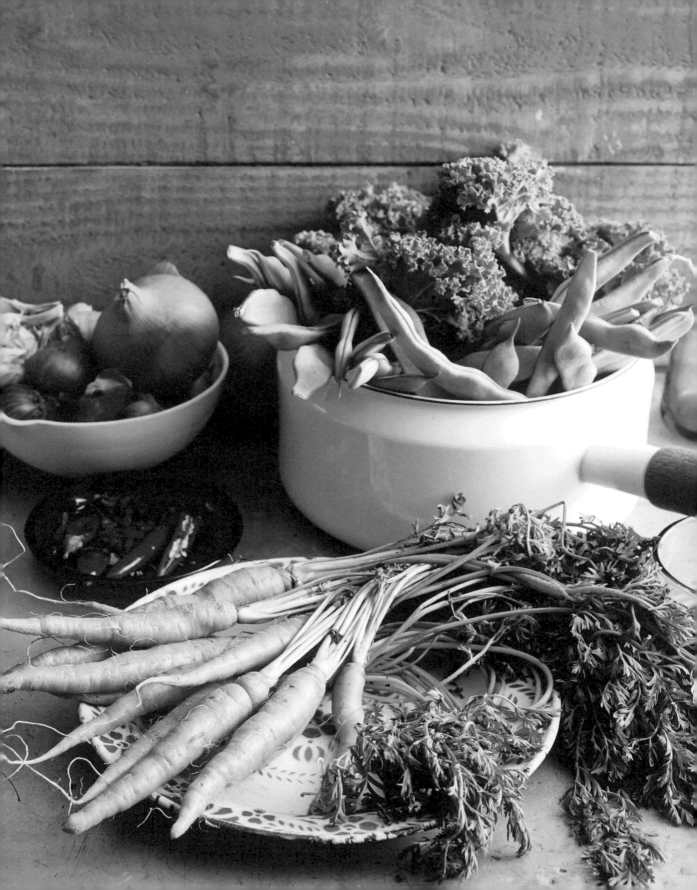

CHAPTER THREE

The Meal Plan

Switching to a new diet can be like moving to a new country. Consider me your tour guide, as I have taken the guesswork out of the planning for you. With this preliminary meal plan, even the pantry and shopping lists are provided to get you started and ready to cook. Just follow along and get ready to prepare some great renal-friendly dishes.

The meal plan and the recipes in this book are designed around busy schedules, like yours may be. Most of the meals are very quick and easy, and there are plenty of grab-and-go options to accommodate the most hectic modern workday. You probably don't want to spend hours in the kitchen, and that's understandable. Who does, after a hard day's work? Many of the meals take just 30 minutes to prepare from start to finish, leaving you with plenty of time to eat right and still live your life.

Pantry List

A pantry list will help you get organized. Stocking the following items in your pantry will make recipe preparation easier and more streamlined. I sometimes suggest a variety of certain items, like noodles, nut butters, oils, and vinegars; however, you don't need to stock all of the varieties listed if you don't want to. For example, some people prefer to keep one kind of nut butter or noodle on hand and use that for all of their recipes. That's totally fine, especially if you're trying to keep your budget and shopping list trim. Note that the week 1 through week 4 shopping lists do not include these pantry items, as it is assumed that you will have them on hand. If you don't want to buy them all at once, you can look over the specific recipes to see which items you'll need for each week.

Have some leftover vegetables? Freeze them for a future meal! For added convenience, label the container with the date, produce variety, and measurement (such as ¼ cup basil or 1 red pepper, sliced).

- Almond butter
- Baking soda
- Barley
- Bulgur
- Black peppercorns
- Bread crumbs, coarse
- Cardamom, ground
- Chia seeds
- Chipotle pepper, ground
- Cinnamon, ground
- Cinnamon, stick
- Cloves, ground
- Cocoa powder
- Coriander, ground
- Coriander, seeds
- Cornmeal, yellow
- Cornstarch
- Couscous

- Cumin, ground
- Cumin, seeds
- Curry powder
- Cream of tartar
- Fennel seeds, ground
- Flaxseed, ground
- Flour, all-purpose
- Flour, buckwheat
- Garam masala
- Garlic powder
- Gelatin powder
- Ginger, ground
- Graham cracker crumbs
- Honey
- Lentils, brown
- Mustard, Dijon
- Nonstick cooking spray
- Noodles, chow mein
- Noodles, egg
- Noodles, fettuccine
- Noodles, linguine
- Noodles, penne, farfalle, elbow, or rotini
- Noodles, rice vermicelli
- Noodles, spaghetti
- Oil, canola
- Oil, extra-virgin olive
- Oil, toasted sesame
- Onion powder
- Oregano, dried
- Paprika, ground
- Parsley, dried
- Peanut butter
- Rice, basmati
- Rice, long-grain white
- Red chili, flakes
- Rolled oats
- Soy sauce, low-sodium
- Sugar, brown
- Sugar, granulated
- Sugar, powdered
- Sunflower seeds
- Tahini
- Tea, black
- Thyme, dried
- Turmeric, ground
- Vanilla extract
- Vinegar, apple cider
- Vinegar, balsamic
- Vinegar, rice
- Vinegar, white
- Vinegar, white wine
- Walnuts
- Wine, dry cooking
- Wine, rice cooking

Week 1 Shopping List

Canned and bottled items

- Chicken stock, low-sodium (2 quarts), or make Simple Chicken Broth (page 180)
- Rice milk, unsweetened (1 quart), or make Homemade Rice Milk (page 70)
- Vegetable broth, low-sodium (1 pint)
- White beans (1 [15-ounce] can)

Dairy and eggs

- Butter, unsalted (1 stick)
- Eggs (1 dozen)
- Parmesan cheese, grated (1 ounce)
- Yogurt, plain, unsweetened (8 ounces)

Protein

- Chicken, cooked (4 ounces)
- Chicken, thighs, bone-in (6)
- Pork tenderloin (2 pounds)
- Salmon, fillet (1 pound)

Produce

- Arugula (4 ounces)
- Asparagus (1 pound)
- Avocado (1)
- Basil, fresh (2 bunches)
- Basil, Thai (1 bunch)
- Bean sprouts, mung (4 ounces)
- Bell peppers, red (3)
- Blueberries (1 pint)
- Carrots (2)
- Cauliflower (1 head)
- Celery (1 bunch)
- Chard (1 bunch)
- Cilantro, fresh (1 bunch)
- Collard greens (2 bunches)
- Corn (1 ear)
- Cucumber (1)
- Garlic (3 heads)
- Ginger (1 knob)
- Jalapeño (1)
- Lemons (6)
- Limes (3)
- Onions, sweet (2)
- Parsley, fresh (1 bunch)
- Parsnips (2)
- Peach (1)
- Rosemary, fresh (1 bunch)
- Rutabaga, small (1)
- Scallions (1 bunch)
- Spinach (1 bunch)
- Strawberries (1 pint)
- Turnips, small (2)

Week 1 Menu

	BREAKFAST	LUNCH	DINNER
MONDAY	Bulgur Bowl with Strawberries and Walnuts (page 61)	Summer Pasta Salad with White Wine Vinaigrette (page 115)	Chicken Pho (page 102)
TUESDAY	Peach Berry Parfait (page 59)	Chicken Pho (leftovers)	Creamy Pesto Pasta (page 129)
WEDNESDAY	Bulgur Bowl with Strawberries and Walnuts (leftovers)	Summer Pasta Salad with White Wine Vinaigrette (leftovers)	Collard and Rice Stuffed Red Peppers (page 125)
THURSDAY	Green Breakfast Soup (page 58)	Creamy Pesto Pasta (leftovers)	One-Pan Curried Chicken Thighs and Cauliflower (page 152)
FRIDAY	Green Breakfast Soup (leftovers)	Collard and Rice Stuffed Red Peppers (leftovers)	Salmon Burgers (page 140) and Mixed Green Leaf and Citrus Salad (page 109)
SATURDAY	Asparagus Frittata (page 66)	Vegetable Lentil Soup (page 100)	White Bean Veggie Burgers (page 119)
SUNDAY	Buckwheat Pancakes (page 63)	Salmon Burgers (leftovers)	Marinated Pork Tenderloin (page 157) and Roasted Root Vegetables (page 89)

WEEK ONE

SNACK IDEAS *(Ingredients for these recipes are not included in shopping list):*

- Handful of strawberries or blueberries
- Collard Salad Rolls with Peanut Dipping Sauce (page 86)
- Savory Collard Chips (page 83)
- Hard-boiled egg
- Unsalted popcorn

Week 2 Shopping List

Canned and bottled items

- Chicken stock, low-sodium (2 quarts), or make Simple Chicken Broth (page 180)
- Chickpeas (1 [15-ounce] can)
- Rice milk, unsweetened (2 quarts)
- Tomatoes, diced, low-sodium (1 [16-ounce] can)
- Vegetable broth, low-sodium (1 quart)

Dairy and eggs

- Cream cheese (8 ounces)
- Eggs (1 dozen)
- Feta cheese, crumbled (1 ounce)
- Parmesan cheese, shredded (2 ounces)
- Yogurt, plain, unsweetened (1 pint)

Frozen foods

- Ready-made pie crust (1)

Protein

- Chicken breasts, boneless, skinless (4)
- Chicken thighs, boneless, skinless (8 ounces)
- Shrimp, medium (10 ounces)
- Tofu, extra-firm (1 [14-ounce] package)
- Turkey breast, ground, lean (1 pound)

Produce

- Avocado (1)
- Basil, fresh (1 bunch)
- Bean sprouts, mung (4 ounces)
- Beans, green (12 ounces)
- Beet (1)
- Blueberries (1 pint)
- Bok choy (1 head)
- Broccoli (1½ pounds)
- Cabbage, green (1 head)
- Carrots (8)
- Cauliflower (2 heads)
- Celery (1 bunch)
- Chile, green (1)
- Cilantro (1 bunch)
- Cucumber (1)
- Garlic (4 heads)
- Ginger (1 knob)

- Leek (1)
- Lemons (4)
- Lettuce, green leaf (1 head)
- Lettuce, red leaf (1 head)
- Microgreens (3 ounces)
- Onion, red (1)
- Onions, sweet (2)
- Oregano, fresh (1 bunch)
- Parsley, fresh (1 bunch)
- Potato (1)
- Scallions (1 bunch)
- Spinach, baby (6 ounces)
- Strawberries (1 pint)

- Thyme, fresh (1 bunch)
- Tomatoes (4)

Other

- Bagel, multigrain (1)

- Tortillas (4)

Week 2 Menu

	BREAKFAST	LUNCH	DINNER
MONDAY	Avocado Egg Bake (page 64)	Creamy Broccoli Soup (page 94)	Spinach Falafel Wrap (page 120)
TUESDAY	Strawberry Cheesecake Smoothie (page 77)	Spinach Falafel Wrap (leftovers)	Turkey Burger Soup (page 103)
WEDNESDAY	Overnight Oats, Chocolate Peanut Butter variety (page 62)	Creamy Broccoli Soup (leftovers)	Chicken Chow Mein (page 146)
THURSDAY	Open-Faced Bagel Breakfast Sandwich (page 60)	Turkey Burger Soup (leftovers)	Cauliflower and Potato Curry (page 118) and rice
FRIDAY	Overnight Oats, Chocolate Peanut Butter variety (leftovers)	Chicken Chow Mein (leftovers)	Creamy Shrimp Fettuccine (page 135)
SATURDAY	Broccoli Basil Quiche (page 65)	Tofu and Rice Salad Bowl (page 123)	Chicken Breast and Bok Choy in Parchment (page 151)
SUNDAY	Poached Eggs with Cilantro Butter (page 67)	Creamy Shrimp Fettuccine (leftovers)	Vegetable Biriyani (page 124)

SNACK IDEAS *(Ingredients for these recipes are not included in shopping list):*

- Strawberries or blueberries with yogurt
- Celery with almond butter or cream cheese
- Cauliflower florets with Thai-Style Eggplant Dip (page 85)
- Cinnamon Apple Chips (page 82)
- Cucumber slices

WEEK TWO

Week 3 Shopping List

Canned and bottled items

- Beef broth, low-sodium (1 pint)
- Black beans (1 [15-ounce] can)
- Chicken stock, low-sodium (2 quarts), or make Simple Chicken Broth (page 180)
- Rice milk, unsweetened (2 quarts), or make Homemade Rice Milk (page 70)
- Vegetable broth, low-sodium (1 pint)

Dairy and eggs

- Butter, unsalted (1 stick)
- Eggs (1 dozen)
- Parmesan cheese, shredded (1 ounce)
- Yogurt, plain, unsweetened (1 pint)

Protein

- Beef, ground, lean (1½ pounds)
- Chicken breast, boneless, skinless (1¾ pounds)
- Halibut, fillet (1 pound)
- Salmon, fillet (1 pound)

Produce

- Arugula (2 ounces)
- Asparagus (1 pound)
- Avocado (1)
- Beans, green (4 ounces)
- Bell pepper, red or yellow (1)
- Beet (1)
- Blueberries (1 pint)
- Broccoli, florets (18 ounces)
- Carrots (6)
- Celery (1 bunch)
- Chiles, Thai red (2)
- Cilantro, fresh (1 bunch)
- Collard greens (1 bunch)
- Corn (1 ear)
- Cucumbers (3)
- Garlic (2 heads)
- Ginger (1 knob)
- Kale (1 bunch)
- Lemongrass, stalk (1)
- Lemons (5)
- Lettuce, green leaf (1 head)
- Limes (2)
- Mint, fresh (1 bunch)
- Mushrooms, cremini (8 ounces)

- Mustard greens (1 bunch)
- Onions, sweet (2)
- Oranges, mandarin (3)
- Parsley, fresh (1 bunch)
- Peach (1)
- Radishes (1 bunch)
- Rosemary, fresh (1 bunch)
- Scallions (1 bunch)
- Shallots (2)
- Spinach (1 bunch)
- Spinach, baby (6 ounces)
- Squash, delicata (2)
- Thyme, fresh (1 bunch)
- Tomatoes, cherry (1 pint)
- Zucchini (3)

Other

- Flatbreads, white (4)
- White bread (1 slice)

Week 3 Menu

	BREAKFAST	LUNCH	DINNER
MONDAY	Peach Berry Parfait (page 59)	Curried Carrot and Beet Soup (page 95) and Spinach Salad with Orange Vinaigrette (page 108)	Chicken Kebab Sandwich (page 144)
TUESDAY	Blueberry Burst Smoothie (page 79)	Bulgur and Broccoli Salad (page 114)	Thai-Style Chicken Curry (page 148)
WEDNESDAY	Peach Berry Parfait (leftovers)	Curried Carrot and Beet Soup (leftovers) and Cucumber and Radish Salad (page 107)	Salmon and Kale in Parchment (page 139)
THURSDAY	Green Breakfast Soup (page 58)	Bulgur and Broccoli Salad (leftovers)	Stuffed Delicata Squash Boats with Bulgur and Vegetables (page 127)
FRIDAY	Overnight Oats, Chocolate Peanut Butter variety (page 62)	Thai-Style Chicken Curry (leftovers)	Bulgur and Greens Soup with Soft-Boiled Egg (page 99)
SATURDAY	Asparagus Frittata (page 66)	Stuffed Delicata Squash Boats with Bulgur and Vegetables (leftovers)	Lemon Garlic Halibut (page 136) and Vegetable Couscous (page 90)
SUNDAY	Buckwheat Pancakes (page 63)	Bulgur and Greens Soup with Soft-Boiled Egg (leftovers)	Meatloaf with Mushroom Gravy (page 158) and Celery and Arugula Salad (page 106)

SNACK IDEAS *(Ingredients for these recipes are not included in shopping list):*

- Cherry tomatoes
- Hard-boiled egg
- Green salad with Balsamic Vinaigrette (page 177)

- Roasted Red Pepper Hummus (page 84) with vegetables
- Handful of blueberries or strawberries

Week 4 Shopping List

Canned and bottled items

- Chicken stock, low-sodium (2 quarts), or make Simple Chicken Broth (page 180)
- Rice milk, unsweetened (1 quart), or make Homemade Rice Milk (page 70)

Dairy and eggs

- Butter, unsalted (1 stick)
- Cream cheese (8 ounces)
- Egg (1 dozen)
- Feta cheese, crumbled (1 ounce)
- Parmesan cheese, shredded (2 ounces)
- Yogurt, plain, unsweetened (8 ounces)

Protein

- Chicken breast, boneless, skinless (10 ounces)
- Salmon, fillet (1 pound)
- Shrimp (1 pound)
- Tofu, extra-firm (1 [14-ounce] package)
- Turkey breast, ground, lean (12 ounces)

Produce

- Arugula (4 ounces)
- Asparagus (1 pound)
- Avocado (1)
- Basil, fresh (1 bunch)
- Beans, green (4 ounces)
- Beets (8 small)
- Bell pepper, red (1)
- Blueberries (1 pint)
- Broccoli (1½ pounds)
- Broccoli rabe (1 bunch)
- Cabbage, green (1 head)
- Carrots (4)
- Cauliflower (2 heads)
- Chives, fresh (1 bunch)
- Cilantro, fresh (1 bunch)
- Cucumber (1)
- Eggplants, Thai (2)
- Garlic (3 heads)
- Ginger (1 knob)
- Greens, baby salad (10 ounces)
- Lemons (4)
- Microgreens (3 ounces)
- Onion, red (1)
- Onions, sweet (3)
- Parsley, fresh (2 bunches)
- Peas, sugar snap (5 ounces)
- Rosemary, fresh (1 bunch)
- Scallions (1 bunch)
- Strawberries (1 pint)
- Thyme, fresh (1 bunch)
- Tomato (1)
- Zucchini (2)

Other

- Bagel, multigrain (1)

Week 4 Menu

	BREAKFAST	LUNCH	DINNER
MONDAY	Bulgur Bowl with Strawberries and Walnuts (page 61)	Cauliflower and Chive Soup (page 98) and Roasted Beet Salad (page 110)	Aromatic Chicken and Cabbage Stir-Fry (page 145)
TUESDAY	Open-Faced Bagel Breakfast Sandwich (page 60)	Summer Pasta Salad with White Wine Vinaigrette (page 115)	Roasted Salmon with Herb Gremolata (page 141) and Simple Roasted Broccoli (page 87)
WEDNESDAY	Bulgur Bowl with Strawberries and Walnuts (leftovers)	Aromatic Chicken and Cabbage Stir-Fry (leftovers)	Barley and Roasted Vegetable Bowl (page 128)
THURSDAY	Overnight Oats, Chocolate Peanut Butter variety (page 62)	Cauliflower and Chive Soup (leftovers) and Summer Pasta Salad with White Wine Vinaigrette (leftovers)	Shrimp Fried Rice (page 134)
FRIDAY	Strawberry Cheesecake Smoothie (page 77)	Shrimp Fried Rice (leftovers)	Turkey Meatballs and Spaghetti in Garlic Sauce (page 155)
SATURDAY	Avocado Egg Bake (page 64)	Asparagus Lemon Soup (page 97)	Vegetable Biriyani (page 124)
SUNDAY	Poached Eggs with Cilantro Butter (page 67)	Asparagus Lemon Soup (leftovers)	Spicy Tofu and Broccoli Stir-Fry (page 121)

SNACK IDEAS *(Ingredients for these recipes are not included in shopping list):*

- Red bell pepper strips
- Cauliflower florets
- Blueberries and yogurt
- Collard Salad Rolls with Peanut Dipping Sauce (page 86)
- Cinnamon Apple Chips (page 82)

WEEK FOUR

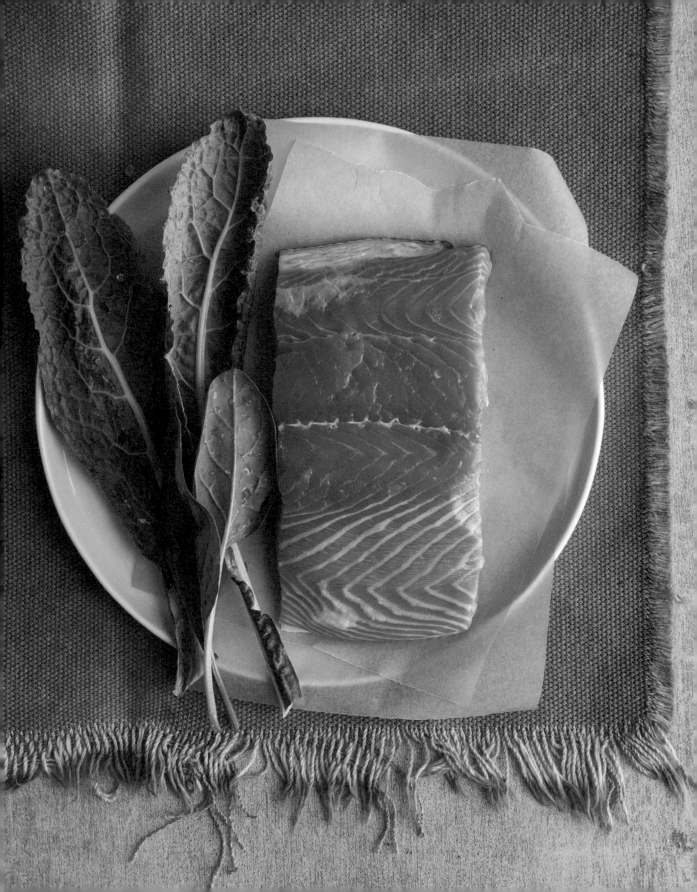

CHAPTER FOUR

A Kidney-Friendly Lifestyle

I am very excited that you have made the choice to learn more about your kidney disease and what you need for optimum health. In this chapter, we will continue down the path to healthy eating with some tips and tools for success. You will learn how to make smart food choices that will allow you to take control of your kidney disease while enjoying life. I am confident your journey to kidney health will be a positive one, as you learn about nutrition and how it impacts your health, and discover all the great foods you can enjoy. By the end of this chapter, you will have all the tools you need to get started. Just keep an open mind and don't be too hard on yourself, because some days will be easy, and others will be more challenging—it's okay! We all have our good and bad days; just remember, it's what you do most days that makes the difference.

Tips for Success

1 ***Be your own best health advocate.*** Don't be afraid to ask questions—lots of them. The more you know, the more control you'll have over your health. The choices you make are the best predictors of your health outcomes, so make informed ones.

2 ***Choose wisely.*** Right, wrong, or indifferent, your outcomes are dependent on the choices you make. Planning is key to avoiding impulsive decisions, so integrate planning into every facet of your diet for best success. Plan meals ahead, keep healthy on-the-go snacks at arm's reach, and don't go food shopping hungry.

3 ***Practice meal planning.*** To streamline the process, follow the weekly grocery lists, especially at first. As you become comfortable with this diet, you'll be able to customize your own meal schedule that balances your preferences with the nutrients you need.

4 ***Fresh is best.*** Processed foods contain unwanted sodium and phosphorus. Cook from fresh, unprocessed whole ingredients to make renal-friendly meals.

5 ***No one is perfect.*** Don't be too hard on yourself. We all have good and bad days, and diet slipups may happen. A thought worth repeating: It's not about perfection but what you do most of the time that matters.

WORKSHEET: Make Your Own Weekly Menu

Use this blank chart to prepare your own weekly menus:

	BREAKFAST	LUNCH	SNACK	DINNER
MONDAY				
TUESDAY				
WEDNESDAY				
THURSDAY				
FRIDAY				
SATURDAY				
SUNDAY				

Dining Out

Going out to eat is fun—and yes, you still can do it! When you have kidney disease, you can dine out without worry if you make smart food choices. Unfortunately, many restaurants add a lot of sodium to their foods, making some dishes unhealthy for just about anyone. With kidney disease, you should be a little more cautious, and watch out for foods that have hidden contents of protein, sodium, potassium, and phosphorus. Along with the tips listed here, use the chart "Strategies for Dining Out" (page 52) to help you make healthier restaurant food choices.

Preview the menu. Many restaurants post menus on their websites—check them out before you go.

Choose the venue. Pick a restaurant where it will be easiest to select foods best suited for your diet, such as one where food is made to order.

Seek answers. Ask your server for more detail about items you don't understand.

Split a meal. Consider sharing a main dish with your dining companion.

Sauce on the side. Ask for salad dressings, gravies, or sauces to be served on the side.

Pass the salt. For any grilled, sautéed, or baked entrées, ask that no salt be added. For Asian foods, ask for no MSG (monosodium glutamate).

Simplify sandwiches. Order sandwiches or burgers without cheese, and ask for mustard or ketchup on the side.

Cut the meat. To scale back on protein, you may want to request half portions of main dishes that contain meat, poultry, fish, or even cheese.

Take it home. Bring part of your main dish home in a takeout box.

Watch for culprits. Keep in mind, protein is found in cheese and cream sauces; food prepared with milk, nuts, and eggs; and vegetarian dishes containing dried beans or lentils.

Social Gatherings

Social events, such as birthdays, weddings, graduations, picnics, and barbecues, are wonderful opportunities to get together and celebrate with family and friends. Let's talk about how to avoid overindulging and instead how to make healthier choices about what to eat and drink that won't leave you feeling deprived. Here are some tips:

Don't go hungry. Try not to leave the house on an empty stomach. Going to any event hungry will set you up for disaster and most likely lead to impulsive overeating. Grab a high-protein snack beforehand, such as a boiled egg with crackers, to help you feel a little full and avoid desperate decisions at the buffet.

Avoid high-sodium foods. Salty foods will make you thirsty, which will make you want to drink more than is recommended. Instead of hot dogs or sausages, seek out lower-sodium foods, such as chicken and hamburgers. Enjoy the barbecue sauce and salad dressing on the side to better control portion sizes, because they are very high in salt. If possible, ask for vegetables to be grilled.

Practice food safety. Kidney disease puts you at higher risk for food-borne illnesses. If you're hosting or assisting with the event, cook food to safe temperatures, wash produce well, and use separate cutting boards for raw and cooked meats.

Plan ahead. Feel free to ask your host about the menu in advance. This way you can decide exactly what you want to eat. If it's not to your liking or doesn't fit with your diet, bring your own dish to share.

Avoid smoking. Smoking can affect medicines used to treat high blood pressure, which is the leading cause of kidney disease. Smoking also slows the blood flow to your kidneys and can even worsen your kidney disease.

Limit alcohol. Alcohol can also affect certain high-blood-pressure medications. Check with your doctor to make sure it is safe for you to drink alcohol.

Focus on folks. Move away from the buffet, and make loved ones the center of your attention.

Strategies for Dining Out

TYPE OF FOOD	AVOID/LIMIT	BETTER CHOICES
BUFFET	Soups (generally high in sodium and potassium); chips, potato wedges, roasted or baked potatoes; raw spinach; olives; pickles; bacon bits; tomatoes; mushrooms; broccoli; kidney beans; seeds or nuts; croutons; potato salad; three-bean salad; olive salads; relishes; pickles; dried fruit; fresh fruit salad; kiwifruit; melons; bananas; oranges	Salad bar (limit serving size to that of a bread and butter plate or a small bowl): lettuce, carrots, radishes, cauliflower, green peppers, celery, onions, cucumbers, green peas, beets, alfalfa sprouts, Chinese noodles, grated cheese (in moderation), coleslaw, macaroni salad, gelatin salads, cottage cheese, canned peaches or pears, canned fruit cocktail, fresh grapes, fresh or canned pineapple, small fresh peach Grilled, pan-fried, or marinated meats; chicken; fish; seafood
ASIAN	Nuts; green leafy vegetables such as bok choy, Chinese spinach, and Chinese cabbage; fried rice; soy sauce; teriyaki sauce	Egg rolls, dim sum, pot stickers Steamed veggies, rice, plain noodles (lower-fat choices) Request that your food be prepared without soy sauce, fish sauce, or monosodium glutamate (MSG), all of which contain a lot of salt
FAST FOOD	French fries (high in potassium), fried fish, fried chicken, ketchup, mustard, milkshakes, dark sodas	Unsalted onion rings (as a substitute for French fries) Salads, when available Ask that condiments be left on the side Burger King: plain hamburger McDonalds: plain hamburger Taco Bell: taco with few or no tomatoes Wendy's: plain single hamburger or grilled-chicken sandwich
MEXICAN	Beans, guacamole, cheese, tomatoes	Plain rice, tacos, burritos, fajitas, and enchiladas filled with minced meat, beef, or chicken Best to order from the à la carte menu

TYPE OF FOOD	AVOID/LIMIT	BETTER CHOICES
ITALIAN	Red sauces (usually high in potassium), white sauces (usually high in phosphorus)	Plain or meat-filled pasta (e.g., spaghetti, fettuccine, penne, tortellini, ravioli) Wine sauces like in chicken marsala Order sauce on the side Small portion (3 ounces) of clam and mussel sauces that are not tomato- or cream-based (better choices than red or white sauces) Salad, bread, very plain pasta, such as garlic and butter pasta One tablespoon of grated Parmesan cheese may be used for added flavor
MEDITERRANEAN	Spinach-filled phyllo pastries, sausage rolls and chiko rolls (very high in sodium), tabouleh, falafel, scalloped potatoes	Cream or white-wine sauces; grilled, pan-fried, or marinated meats, chicken, fish, or seafood; dishes served with rice; couscous; kebabs and skewered lean meats; risotto
BARBECUE	Barbecue sauce, steak sauce, mustard, ketchup, horseradish, sausage, hot dogs, corn bread	Lean meat, chicken, fish, or seafood; French bread or garlic bread; grilled vegetables Marinades with wine, lemon juice, oil, vinegar, garlic, honey, herbs, and spices
ENTRÉES	Casseroles; sauces; gravies; heavily fried items; breaded or battered foods; cured or salted meats; omelets with cheese, ham, sausage, or bacon	Broiled or grilled lean meats and fish, omelets with vegetables, sandwiches with meat filling
SIDES	Kale, spinach, potatoes or potato salad, tomatoes, mushrooms, winter squash, baked or fried beans, sauerkraut, vegetables in heavy creams or sauces	Peas, sweet peas, green beans, corn, cabbage, zucchini, eggplant, cauliflower, lentils; plain rice, jasmine rice, pastas, noodles
DESSERT	Chocolate; nuts; coconut; cheesecake; custard; puddings; dried fruit, star fruit, cantaloupe, oranges; pies such as cream, minced, pumpkin, rhubarb, and pecan; ice cream	Low-potassium fresh fruit or canned fruit, sugar cookies, angel food cake, gelatin

Working Through Slipups

Adjusting to a new diet and lifestyle can be difficult—after all, you're creating new habits. Slipups happen, and you will actually have more success if you don't beat yourself up when you veer off track. I want to share some self-compassion strategies that will help you work through your slipups with grace. These tactics can also help you understand and process some of the emotions that you may be experiencing.

- *Embrace your humanity.* Perfection doesn't exist, and expecting perfection paves the way for a big letdown. So if you've stumbled, use this as an opportunity to accept and welcome the fact that you're human.
- *Give thanks to your failures.* Learn from your experience, instead of feeling guilty. You'll gain valuable wisdom and perspective from the experience of disappointment and the resolve of trying to do better.
- *Commit to grow.* Accept that this letdown was the stimulus you needed to cement your commitment to healthier habits and wean away from bad ones. Take this opportunity to reflect, and commit to whatever action it takes to grow from your slipup.
- *Be kind to yourself.* It's okay if you turned to junk food. It's done—graciously accept that reality, give yourself a hug, and move on.

Rest, Relaxation, and Activity

Some days we all feel a little overwhelmed. With a new chronic-kidney-disease diagnosis, you may be dealing with high stress levels. It's important to both your physical and your emotional health to maintain healthy stress levels, so you'll want to find ways to maintain a sense of calm, and with a few lifestyle adjustments, you can arm yourself with what you need for your mind and body to function at their best. Rest and relaxation are enjoyable pursuits, but they're also rituals that your body needs in order to recharge and regroup for busy days and healthy living. Additionally, physical activity is more important than ever when you have kidney disease. For starters, statistics reveal the number one cause of death in patients with kidney disease is related to heart disease. But 30 minutes of exercise a day may help curb those cardiovascular predispositions. In fact, physical activity of any kind can help with blood circulation, reducing stress, boosting energy levels, building strong muscles, sleeping better, and weight management. So carve out time to walk, swim, meditate—whatever works best for you.

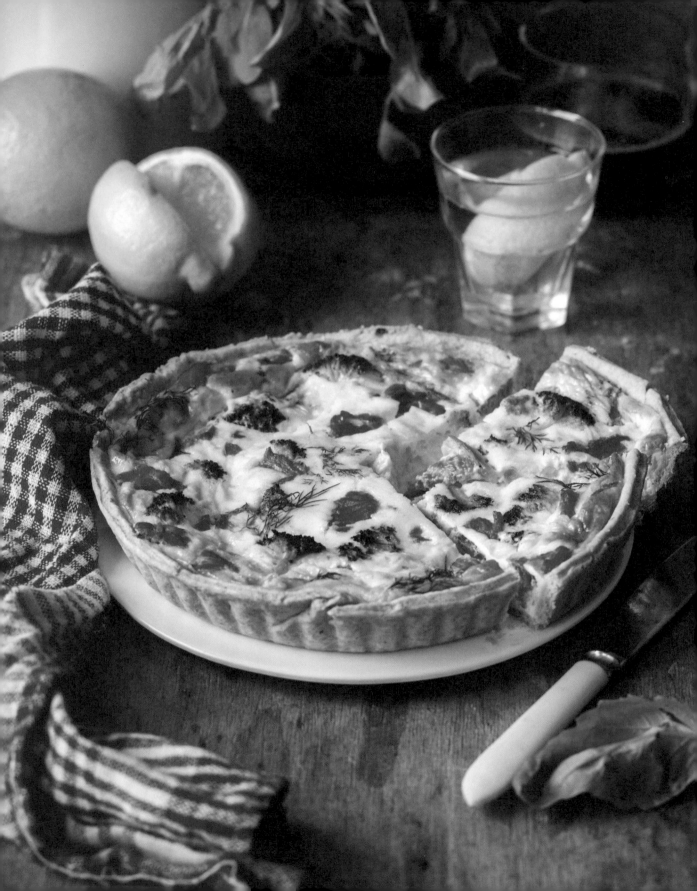

CHAPTER FIVE

Breakfast

◀ *Broccoli Basil Quiche, page 65*

Green Breakfast Soup

SERVES 2 • PREP TIME: 5 MINUTES • COOK TIME: 5 MINUTES

Mealtime is so important, and ideally we ought to sit and enjoy each and every meal. In today's hectic world, though, sometimes things can get rushed, especially breakfast on a busy morning. This soup is actually perfect for such a day. Make it quickly on the stove and transfer it to your to-go mug, and sip this nutrient-rich soup on your morning commute.

2 cups spinach

1 avocado, halved

2 cups low-sodium vegetable or chicken broth (see Lower sodium tip)

1 teaspoon ground coriander

1 teaspoon ground cumin

1 teaspoon ground turmeric

Freshly ground black pepper

1 In a blender or food processor, add the spinach, avocado, broth, coriander, cumin, and turmeric. Process until smooth.

2 Transfer the mixture to a small saucepan over medium heat, and cook until heated through, 2 to 3 minutes. Season with pepper.

Lower sodium tip: *If you want to lower the sodium further, consider making your own Simple Chicken Broth (page 180) for more control over the ingredients. Freeze the broth in 2-cup portions so you can make quick soups when needed.*

Per Serving Calories: 221; Total Fat: 18g; Saturated Fat: 3g; Cholesterol: 0mg; Carbohydrates: 15g; Fiber: 10g; Protein: 5g; Phosphorus: 58mg; Potassium: 551mg; Sodium: 170mg

Peach Berry Parfait

SERVES 2 • PREP TIME: 5 MINUTES

This parfait is like summer in a cup. Blueberries and peaches add natural sweetness to the parfait, while walnuts provide a little added protein and an enjoyable crunch. Walnuts are a great source of omega-3s, plus, according to traditional Chinese medicine, they are thought to help tonify and strengthen the kidneys. Because they are high in potassium, enjoying them in moderation is key.

1 cup plain, unsweetened
   yogurt, divided

1 teaspoon vanilla extract

1 small peach, diced

½ cup blueberries

2 tablespoons
   walnut pieces

1　In a small bowl, mix together the yogurt and vanilla. Add 2 tablespoons of yogurt to each of 2 cups. Divide the diced peach and the blueberries between the cups, and top with the remaining yogurt.

2　Sprinkle each cup with 1 tablespoon of walnut pieces.

Cooking tip: Make these up to three days in advance, cover, and refrigerate until ready to eat.

Per Serving Calories: 191; Total Fat: 10g; Saturated Fat: 3g; Cholesterol: 15mg; Carbohydrates: 14g; Fiber: 14g; Protein: 12g; Phosphorus: 189mg; Potassium: 327mg; Sodium: 40mg

Open-Faced Bagel Breakfast Sandwich

SERVES 2 • PREP TIME: 5 MINUTES • COOK TIME: 5 MINUTES

Enjoy this breakfast bagel on a lazy morning or when you need a quick breakfast on the go. Stacked with fresh vegetables, this simple open-faced sandwich may be just what you need to brighten a dark morning. Play around with different types of microgreens until you find one you really like. Spicy blends can be fun for a sandwich like this, or use baby salad greens for something milder.

1 multigrain bagel, halved

2 tablespoons cream
    cheese, divided

2 slices tomato

1 slice red onion

Freshly ground
    black pepper

1 cup microgreens

1 In a toaster or oven, lightly toast the bagel.

2 Spread 1 tablespoon of cream cheese on each of the bagel halves, and top each half with 1 slice of tomato and a couple rings of onion. Season with the black pepper. Top each half with ½ cup of microgreens and serve.

Substitution tip: *Swap out the red onion for scallions or chives, the tomato for red bell pepper strips, or the microgreens for sprouts as needed to fit what you have on hand. You can also substitute the cream cheese with feta or Brie; just be sure to keep the portion size around 1 tablespoon per serving.*

Per Serving Calories: 156; Total Fat: 6g; Saturated Fat: 3g; Cholesterol: 18mg; Carbohydrates: 22g; Fiber: 3g; Protein: 5g; Protein: 5g; Phosphorus: 98mg; Potassium: 163mg; Sodium: 195mg

Bulgur Bowl with Strawberries and Walnuts

SERVES 4 • PREP TIME: 10 MINUTES • COOK TIME: 15 MINUTES

Fans of oatmeal will love this bulgur bowl just bursting with flavor. Bulgur results from steaming, drying, crushing, and removing the bran from whole-wheat berries, leaving you with a whole grain that is lower in phosphorus and potassium than most whole grains, so it supports your kidneys.

1 cup bulgur

1 cup strawberries, sliced

4 tablespoons (¼ cup) Homemade Rice Milk (page 70) or unsweetened store-bought rice milk

4 teaspoons brown sugar

4 teaspoons extra-virgin olive oil

4 tablespoons (¼ cup) walnut pieces

4 tablespoons (¼ cup) cacao nibs (optional)

1 In a small pot, combine the bulgur with 2 cups of water. Bring to a boil, then lower the heat and let simmer, covered, for 12 to 15 minutes, until tender. Remove from the heat and drain any excess water.

2 In each of four bowls, add a quarter of the bulgur and top with ¼ cup of strawberries, 1 tablespoon of rice milk, 1 teaspoon of brown sugar, 1 teaspoon of olive oil, 1 tablespoon of walnut pieces, and 1 tablespoon of cacao nibs (if using).

Cooking tip: Bulgur can be made up to five days in advance and stored in an airtight container in the refrigerator. To serve, heat in the microwave or, on a warm day, serve cold for a refreshing breakfast bowl.

Per Serving Calories: 190; Total Fat: 9g; Saturated Fat: 1g; Cholesterol: 0mg; Carbohydrates: 26g; Fiber: 5g; Protein: 4g; Phosphorus: 66mg; Potassium: 153mg; Sodium: 13mg

Overnight Oats Three Ways

SERVES 2 • PREP TIME: 5 MINUTES

Simple-to-make overnight oats take the cooking out of mealtime. This mix-and-go recipe is best prepared the night before, or up to three days in advance. The cold version is refreshing, but if you prefer a hot bowl of oats, heat the prepared oatmeal in the microwave before serving.

¾ cup Homemade Rice Milk (page 70) or unsweetened store-bought rice milk

½ cup plain, unsweetened yogurt

½ cup rolled oats

1 tablespoon ground flaxseed

1 teaspoon vanilla extract

2 teaspoons honey

VARIATION 1: CHOCOLATE PEANUT BUTTER

2 tablespoons natural unsalted peanut butter

2 tablespoons cocoa powder

VARIATION 2: BLUEBERRY CHEESECAKE

¼ cup blueberries

2 tablespoons cream cheese, at room temperature

Zest and juice of ½ lemon

1 In a medium bowl, mix the rice milk, yogurt, oats, flaxseed, vanilla, and honey.

2 Add the ingredients to make your preferred variation, and stir to blend.

3 Divide between two jars, cover, and refrigerate for at least 4 hours or overnight.

Substitution tip: These oats can be flavored to suit your tastes. Strawberries, raspberries, blackberries, and peaches all go well with oats. For an extra nutritional boost, try adding a small handful of unsalted nuts, or a teaspoon of chia seeds or hemp seeds to your bowl.

Per Serving (plain) Calories: 196; Total Fat: 7g; Saturated Fat: 2g; Cholesterol: 7mg; Carbohydrates: 25g; Fiber: 3g; Protein: 8g; Phosphorus: 99mg; Potassium: 114mg; Sodium: 63mg

Per Serving (Chocolate Peanut Butter) Calories: 299; Total Fat: 15g; Saturated Fat: 4g; Cholesterol: 7mg; Carbohydrates: 31g; Fiber: 6g; Protein: 13g; Phosphorus: 139mg; Potassium: 196mg; Sodium: 69mg

Per Serving (Blueberry Cheesecake) Calories: 259; Total Fat: 12g; Saturated Fat: 5g; Cholesterol: 23mg; Carbohydrates: 30g; Fiber: 3g; Protein: 9g; Phosphorus: 118mg; Potassium: 160mg; Sodium: 109mg

Buckwheat Pancakes

SERVES 4 • PREP TIME: 10 MINUTES • COOK TIME: 15 MINUTES

Made from unroasted buckwheat groats, buckwheat flour lends pancakes a rich, nutty flavor. White flour keeps them tender and light like a pancake should be, and baking powder provides the cakes with a nice lift. Top them with strawberries or blueberries and a sprinkle of powdered sugar, and you'll have a whole-grain breakfast that's yummy and filling.

1¾ cups Homemade Rice Milk (page 70) or unsweetened store-bought rice milk

2 teaspoons white vinegar

1 cup buckwheat flour

½ cup all-purpose flour

1 tablespoon sugar

2 teaspoons Phosphorus-Free Baking Powder (page 174)

1 large egg

1 teaspoon vanilla extract

2 tablespoons butter, for the skillet

1 In a small bowl, combine the rice milk and vinegar. Let sit for 5 minutes.

2 Meanwhile, in a large bowl, mix the buckwheat flour and all-purpose flour. Add the sugar and baking powder, stirring to blend.

3 Add the egg and vanilla to the rice milk and stir to blend. Add the wet ingredients to the dry, and stir until just mixed.

4 In a large skillet over medium heat, melt 1½ teaspoons of butter. Use a ¼-cup measuring cup to scoop the batter into the skillet. Cook for 2 to 3 minutes, until small bubbles form on the surface of the pancakes. Flip and cook on the opposite side for 1 to 2 minutes.

5 Transfer the pancakes to a serving platter, and in batches, continue cooking the remaining batter in the skillet, adding more butter as needed.

Lower sodium tip: There are several low-sodium and no-sodium baking powders on the market, but they can be hard to find in grocery stores. If you need to lower your sodium further, purchase low-sodium or no-sodium baking powder online.

Per Serving Calories: 264; Total Fat: 9g; Saturated Fat: 3g; Cholesterol: 58mg; Carbohydrates: 39g; Fiber: 3g; Protein: 7g; Phosphorus: 147mg; Potassium: 399mg; Sodium: 232mg

Avocado Egg Bake

SERVES 2 • PREP TIME: 5 MINUTES • COOK TIME: 15 MINUTES

Avocados are a wonderful source of monounsaturated fatty acids, B vitamins, vitamin E, and fiber. Start your day right by combining this powerful and nutrient-dense fruit with an egg for a filling meal. Look for an avocado that yields gently to pressure when holding, but avoid using an overly ripe avocado—it needs to remain slightly firm during cooking.

1 avocado, halved

2 large eggs

Freshly ground
  black pepper

1 tablespoon
  chopped parsley

1 Preheat the oven to 425°F.

2 In a small bowl, crack 1 egg carefully, keeping the yolk intact.

3 On a baking sheet, place the avocado halves cut-side up. Pour the egg into one half. Repeat with the other egg and avocado half. Season with pepper.

4 Bake for 15 minutes, until the egg is set. Remove from the oven, and sprinkle with the parsley. Serve.

Substitution tip: For new flavor combinations, experiment with different herbs on top of the finished egg bake. Cilantro, chives, scallions, and fresh oregano are other lively flavors to top off this dish.

Per Serving Calories: 242; Total Fat: 20g; Saturated Fat: 4g; Cholesterol: 208mg; Carbohydrates: 9g; Fiber: 7g; Protein: 9g; Phosphorus: 164mg; Potassium: 575mg; Sodium: 88mg

Broccoli Basil Quiche

SERVES 8 • PREP TIME: 10 MINUTES • COOK TIME: 55 MINUTES

Quiche is a classic breakfast comfort food. In this reworked, healthier version, we've lowered the fat from the amount in a traditional quiche made with—and achieved this without in the least compromising flavor. Make this up to two days in advance and reheat before serving. Serve the quiche with a side of fresh berries for a meal that will power you through your morning.

1 store-bought
   frozen piecrust
2 cups finely
   chopped broccoli
1 tomato, chopped
2 scallions, chopped
3 eggs, beaten
2 tablespoons
   chopped basil
1 cup Homemade
   Rice Milk (page 70)
   or unsweetened
   store-bought rice milk
½ cup crumbled
   feta cheese
1 garlic clove, minced
1 tablespoon
   all-purpose flour
Freshly ground
   black pepper

1 Preheat the oven to 425°F.

2 Line a pie pan with the piecrust, and use a fork to pierce the crust in several places. Bake the crust for 10 minutes. Remove from the oven and reduce the temperature to 325°F.

3 In a medium bowl, mix the broccoli, tomato, scallions, eggs, basil, rice milk, feta, garlic, and flour. Season with pepper.

4 Pour the broccoli-and-egg mixture into the prepared pie pan. Bake for 35 to 45 minutes, until a knife inserted in the center comes out clean. Let cool for 10 to 15 minutes before serving.

Lower sodium tip: *To reduce the sodium even further, omit the crust. Instead, spray the pan with nonstick cooking spray and bake as directed. This will cut the sodium in the dish to 157mg.*

Per Serving Calories: 160; Total Fat: 10g; Saturated Fat: 3g; Cholesterol: 87mg; Carbohydrates: 13g; Fiber: 1g; Protein: 6g; Phosphorus: 101mg; Potassium: 173mg; Sodium: 259mg

Asparagus Frittata

SERVES 2 • PREP TIME: 5 MINUTES • COOK TIME: 30 MINUTES

A frittata, similar to an omelet, can take on whatever vegetables and seasonings you throw at it. Roasted asparagus is the star of this one-dish wonder with its unique flavor and tender appeal. Soothing to the body, asparagus helps energize the kidneys, making it a great vegetable to start the day. Because it's not commercially grown with pesticides, you can skip the organic variety, and instead look for stalks of uniform size for even cooking. Roast the asparagus the night before, while you're making dinner, to expedite preparation in the morning.

10 medium asparagus
    spears, ends trimmed

2 teaspoons extra-virgin
    olive oil, divided

Freshly ground
    black pepper

4 large eggs

½ teaspoon onion powder

¼ cup chopped parsley

1 Preheat the oven to 450°F.

2 Toss the asparagus with 1 teaspoon of olive oil and season with pepper. Transfer to a baking pan and roast, stirring occasionally, for 20 minutes, until the spears are browned and tender.

3 In a small bowl, beat the eggs with the onion powder and parsley. Season with pepper.

4 Cut the asparagus spears into 1-inch pieces and arrange in a medium skillet. Drizzle with the remaining oil, and shake the pan to distribute.

5 Pour the egg mixture into the skillet, and cook over medium heat. When the egg is well set on the bottom and nearly set on the top, cover it with a plate, invert the pan so the frittata is on the plate, and then slide it back into the pan with the cooked-side up. Continue to cook for about 30 more seconds, until firm.

Substitution tip: For an entirely different flavor, try a veggie frittata with mushrooms, red bell peppers, spinach, or broccoli.

Per Serving Calories: 102; Total Fat: 8g; Saturated Fat: 2g; Cholesterol: 104mg; Carbohydrates: 4g; Fiber: 2g; Protein: 6g; Phosphorus: 103mg; Potassium: 248mg; Sodium: 46mg

Poached Eggs
with Cilantro Butter

SERVES 2 • PREP TIME: 5 MINUTES • COOK TIME: 10 MINUTES

Poached eggs are easy to make with this technique—creating a wonderful breakfast with their creamy yolk and tender whites. Topped with a fragrant herb butter, these eggs go great over a piece of toast, or even on their own.

2 tablespoons
   unsalted butter

1 tablespoon
   chopped parsley

1 tablespoon
   chopped cilantro

4 large eggs

Dash vinegar

Freshly ground
   black pepper

1 In a small pan over low heat, melt the butter. Add the parsley and cilantro, and cook for about 1 minute, stirring constantly. Remove from the heat, and pour into a small dish.

2 In a small saucepan, bring about 3 inches of water to a simmer. Add the dash of vinegar.

3 Crack 1 egg into a cup or ramekin. Using a spoon, create a whirlpool in the simmering water, and then pour the egg into the water. Use the spoon to draw the white together until just starting to set. Repeat with the remaining eggs. Cook for 4 to 7 minutes, depending on how set you like your yolk.

4 With a slotted spoon, remove the eggs.

5 Serve the eggs topped with 1 tablespoon of the herbed butter and some pepper.

Substitution tip: *A light-tasting olive oil can be used in place of butter in this recipe. Loaded with heart-healthy monounsaturated fat, olive oil has a unique flavor that works well to tie together many elements of a meal.*

Ingredient tip: *The vinegar lowers the cooking temperature of the egg, enabling it to solidify sooner.*

Per Serving Calories: 261; Total Fat: 22g; Saturated Fat: 7g; Cholesterol: 429mg; Carbohydrates: 1g; Fiber: 0g; Protein: 14g; Phosphorus: 226mg; Potassium: 173mg; Sodium: 164mg

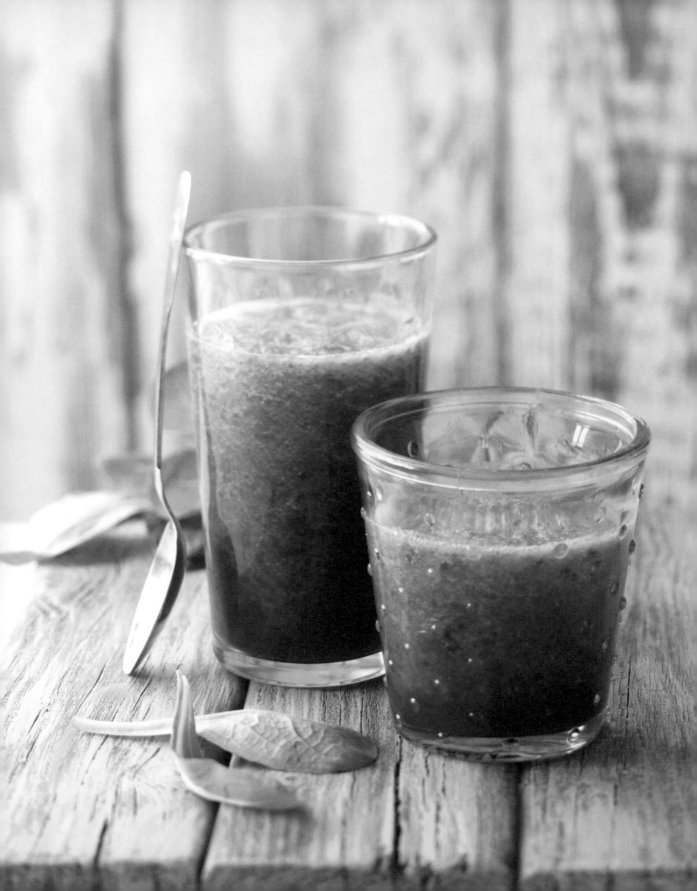

CHAPTER SIX

Smoothies and Drinks

◀ *Cucumber Spinach Green Smoothie, page 78*

Homemade Rice Milk

SERVES 4 • PREP TIME: 5 MINUTES, PLUS 8 TO 12 HOURS TO SOAK

Store-bought milk alternatives can be high in phosphorus and potassium, and because these micronutrients aren't typically included on product labels, and recipes change often, knowing which to buy requires research and diligence. Thankfully, you can easily make rice milk on your own, so you'll know exactly what's in it. To serve on its own or in cereal, add the optional vanilla extract to give the rice milk some extra flavor, but when using rice milk for cooking, it's best to leave it out.

1 cup long-grain white rice

4 cups water

½ teaspoon vanilla extract (optional)

1 In a medium dry skillet over medium heat, toast the rice until lightly browned, about 5 minutes.

2 Transfer the rice to a jar or bowl, and add the water. Cover, refrigerate, and soak overnight.

3 In a blender, add the rice and water, along with the vanilla (if using), and process until smooth.

4 Place a fine-mesh strainer over a glass jar or bowl, and pour the milk into it. Serve immediately, or cover, refrigerate, and serve within three days. Shake before using.

Substitution tip: *Rice milk can be substituted in most recipes calling for whole milk or another nut milk as a low-fat, low-phosphorus, and low-potassium alternative. Use an equal amount of rice milk in place of other milk products, and proceed as directed in the recipe.*

Per Serving Calories: 112; Total Fat: 0g; Saturated Fat: 0g; Cholesterol: 0mg; Carbohydrates: 24g; Fiber: 0g; Protein: 0g; Phosphorus: 0mg; Potassium: 55mg; Sodium: 80mg

Cinnamon Horchata

Horchata, a Mexican drink, is traditionally made with a combination of ground rice, nuts, and seeds. In this simple version, rice stands alone to create a creamy and nourishing beverage that is just right for a hot summer day. Because the horchata must rest for at least three hours, get started on this recipe early if you are expecting company.

1 cup long-grain white rice

4 cups water

1 cinnamon stick,
   broken into pieces

1 cup Homemade
   Rice Milk (page 70)
   or unsweetened
   store-bought rice milk

1 teaspoon vanilla extract

1 teaspoon
   ground cinnamon

⅓ cup granulated sugar

1 In a blender, combine the rice, water, and cinnamon-stick pieces. Blend for about 1 minute, until the rice begins to break up. Let stand at room temperature for at least 3 hours or overnight.

2 Place a wire mesh strainer over a pitcher, and pour the liquid into it. Discard the rice.

3 Add the milk, vanilla, ground cinnamon, and sugar. Stir to combine. Serve over ice.

Variation tip: For an even richer flavor, add 1 tablespoon of unsweetened cocoa powder to the horchata with the ground cinnamon in Step 3.

Per Serving Calories: 123; Total Fat: 2g; Saturated Fat: 0g; Cholesterol: 0mg; Carbohydrates: 26g; Fiber: 0g; Protein: 1g; Phosphorus: 34mg; Potassium: 78mg; Sodium: 32mg

Berry Mint Water

SERVES 8 • PREP TIME: 5 MINUTES, PLUS 1 HOUR TO CHILL

If you're cutting back on soda and struggling with plain water, this infusion may be just what you need to liven things up. Garnish each cup with a couple pieces of fruit, and enjoy the natural sugar rush that this simple drink provides. Once you get the hang of infusing waters, experiment with your favorite fruits to make your own original and beneficial blend.

8 cups water

½ cup strawberries

½ cup blackberries

3 mint sprigs

In a large pitcher, mix the water, strawberries, blackberries, and mint. Cover and chill for at least 1 hour before drinking. Store in the refrigerator for up to two days.

Substitution tip: *Substitute any of your favorite fruits in this recipe to create your own flavored water. You can also try out different herbs to add bold and complementary flavors. Some additional herbs that taste nice paired with fruit include cilantro, basil, rosemary, and thyme. Ginger root is another favorite water flavor enhancer that stimulates digestion and cleanses the kidneys.*

Per Serving Calories: 7; Total Fat: 0g; Saturated Fat: 0g; Cholesterol: 0mg; Carbohydrates: 2g; Fiber: 1g; Protein: 0g; Phosphorus: 4mg; Potassium: 28mg; Sodium: 0mg

Fennel Digestive Cooler

SERVES 2 • PREP TIME: 5 MINUTES • COOK TIME: 15 MINUTES

Fennel, a uniquely flavored flowering plant species, also serves as a digestive aid that is both cooling and delicious. It is woefully underused in the modern kitchen, but you can change that with this simple, refreshing, and energizing drink. Fennel seeds should be green or greenish brown. If you have a jar sitting in your cupboard and the seeds have turned gray, they're past their prime and flavor, and should be replaced.

2 cups Homemade
   Rice Milk (page 70)
   or unsweetened
   store-bought rice milk
¼ cup fennel seeds, ground
¼ teaspoon ground cloves
1 tablespoon honey

1 In a blender, combine the milk, fennel seeds, cloves, and honey. Process until smooth, and let rest for 30 minutes.

2 Pour over a wire mesh strainer lined with cheesecloth or over a coffee filter set over a glass or jar. Serve.

Nutrition tip: *Fennel is a warming herb that is supportive in treating indigestion, gas, and hypertension. High in quercetin, an antioxidant flavonoid, fennel fights inflammation and inhibits the development of cancer, among other benefits.*

Per Serving Calories: 163; Total Fat: 2g; Saturated Fat: 0g; Cholesterol: 0mg; Carbohydrates: 30g; Fiber: 5g; Protein: 3g; Phosphorus: 57mg; Potassium: 205mg; Sodium: 141mg

Mint Lassi

SERVES 2 • PREP TIME: 5 MINUTES

The cooling properties in mint make this drink perfect for a hot afternoon. Originating from the Indian subcontinent, a lassi is a yogurt-based drink seasoned with popular spices from that region, such as cumin, cardamom, and even chiles. If you want a thinner drink, add a bit more water, 1 tablespoon at a time, until the desired consistency is achieved.

1 teaspoon cumin seeds

½ cup mint leaves

1 cup plain, unsweetened yogurt

½ cup water

1 In a dry skillet over medium heat, toast the cumin seeds until fragrant, 1 to 2 minutes.

2 Transfer the seeds to a blender, along with the mint, yogurt, and water, and process until smooth.

Substitution tip: *If you prefer the flavor of cilantro over mint, try it here instead. Another great substitute is to use ½ cup of strawberries along with ¼ teaspoon of ground cardamom in lieu of the mint.*

Per Serving Calories: 114; Total Fat: 6g; Saturated Fat: 3g; Cholesterol: 15mg; Carbohydrates: 5g; Fiber: 0g; Protein: 10g; Phosphorus: 158mg; Potassium: 179mg; Sodium: 43mg

Vanilla Chia Smoothie

SERVES 2 • PREP TIME: 5 MINUTES • COOK TIME: 5 MINUTES

Chai tea is a refreshing blend loaded with warming spices. Cinnamon, ginger, cardamom, and cloves all lend their unique flavors to this iced concoction that will give you the burst of energy to make it through a long morning. Chia seeds thicken the smoothie and add a bit of helpful fiber and protein, providing lasting energy.

1 cup Homemade
  Rice Milk (page 70)
  or unsweetened
  store-bought rice milk

2 black tea bags

1 teaspoon vanilla extract

1 cup ice

1 teaspoon honey

2 tablespoons chia seeds

½ teaspoon
  ground cinnamon

½ teaspoon ground ginger

¼ teaspoon
  ground cardamom

¼ teaspoon ground cloves

1 In a small pan, heat the rice milk to just steaming. Steep the tea bags for 5 minutes, then discard.

2 In a blender, combine the rice milk, vanilla, ice, honey, chia seeds, cinnamon, ginger, cardamom, and cloves. Process until smooth, and serve.

Substitution tip: To make this ahead, complete Step 1 and refrigerate the milk tea in an airtight container. When ready to make the smoothie, proceed as directed, reducing the ice to ½ cup and adding ¼ cup of water.

Per Serving Calories: 143; Total Fat: 5g; Saturated Fat: 1g; Cholesterol: 0mg; Carbohydrates: 19g; Fiber: 6g; Protein: 3g; Phosphorus: 3mg; Potassium: 93mg; Sodium: 73mg

Watermelon Kiwi Smoothie

SERVES 2 • PREP TIME: 5 MINUTES

Nothing says summer like the flavors of watermelon and kiwi. Because both fruits are high in potassium, portion size is important when enjoying these sweet treats. Feel refreshed, and get plenty of vitamin C in the process, drinking this vibrantly colored smoothie.

2 cups watermelon chunks

1 kiwifruit, peeled

1 cup ice

In a blender, combine the watermelon, kiwi, and ice. Process until smooth.

Nutrition tip: *While watermelon tastes particularly sweet, it has only half the sugar of an apple. Because sugar is the main taste-producing element, it stands out the most. The other primary ingredient in watermelon is water.*

Per Serving Calories: 67; Total Fat: 0g; Saturated Fat: 0g; Cholesterol: 0mg; Carbohydrates: 17g; Fiber: 2g; Protein: 1g; Phosphorus: 28mg; Potassium: 278mg; Sodium: 3mg

Strawberry Cheesecake Smoothie

SERVES 2 • PREP TIME: 5 MINUTES

This dessert in a glass tastes every bit as delicious as it sounds. Strawberries emerge in spring, just when we need them most. They serve as an excellent detoxifier and help support the kidneys, liver, and spleen. Loaded with as much vitamin C as oranges, strawberries make a welcome addition to a diet any time of year.

1 cup Homemade
   Rice Milk (page 70)
   or unsweetened
   store-bought rice milk

1 cup strawberries, hulled

2 tablespoons cream
   cheese, at room
   temperature

½ teaspoon honey

1 teaspoon vanilla extract

3 to 5 ice cubes

In a blender, combine the rice milk, strawberries, cream cheese, honey, vanilla, and ice cubes. Process until smooth, and serve.

Substitution tip: Make your own cheesecake smoothie by substituting another favorite fruit for the strawberries. Blackberries, blueberries, and raspberries all work nicely in this treat.

Per Serving Calories: 114; Total Fat: 6g; Saturated Fat: 3g; Cholesterol: 16mg; Carbohydrates: 13g; Fiber: 1g; Protein: 1g; Phosphorus: 33mg; Potassium: 132mg; Sodium: 102mg

Cucumber Spinach Green Smoothie

SERVES 2 • PREP TIME: 5 MINUTES

Green smoothies empower, especially when they have just enough natural sweetness and flavor to make you crave them. This smoothie succeeds, with a nutrient-packed blend of apple and cucumber—cooling and delicious.

½ cucumber, peeled and
   roughly chopped
½ green apple,
   roughly chopped
1 cup Homemade
   Rice Milk (page 70)
   or unsweetened
   store-bought rice milk
2 cups spinach
3 ice cubes

In a blender, combine the cucumber, apple, milk, spinach, and ice. Process until smooth, and serve.

Substitution tip: A tart green apple is lovely in this smoothie, as it creates a subtle sweetness. However, if you prefer, other apples, such as Fuji, Red Delicious, or McIntosh, can be used. If you are using a thick-skinned apple, peel it first for a nicer texture in the finished smoothie.

Per Serving Calories: 75; Total Fat: 2g; Saturated Fat: 0g; Cholesterol: 0mg; Carbohydrates: 14g; Fiber: 2g; Protein: 1g; Phosphorus: 34mg; Potassium: 313mg; Sodium: 81mg

Blueberry Burst Smoothie

SERVES 2 • PREP TIME: 5 MINUTES

Blueberries lend their characteristic sweetness as the backbone of this brightly colored smoothie, while collard greens offer a bitter tone that adds depth. A single tablespoon of almond butter adds so much comforting flavor that this might just become your go-to quick breakfast or on-the-go snack.

1 cup blueberries

1 cup chopped
   collard greens

1 cup Homemade
   Rice Milk (page 70)
   or unsweetened
   store-bought rice milk

1 tablespoon
   almond butter

3 ice cubes

In a blender, combine the blueberries, collard greens, milk, almond butter, and ice cubes. Process until smooth, and serve.

Nutrition tip: Collard greens are a nutrient-dense food loaded with anticarcinogenic, antiviral, antibiotic, and antioxidant properties. Because collard greens are much lower in potassium than kale, they are a great substitute in recipes that call for its cruciferous cousin.

Per Serving Calories: 131; Total Fat: 6g; Saturated Fat: 0g; Cholesterol: 0mg; Carbohydrates: 19g; Fiber: 3g; Protein: 3g; Phosphorus: 51mg; Potassium: 146mg; Sodium: 60mg

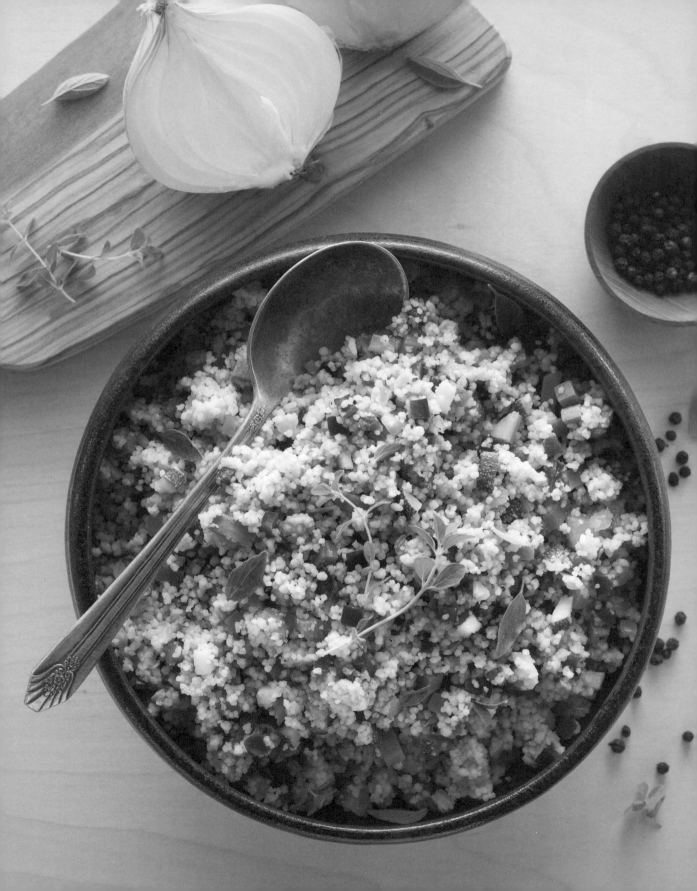

CHAPTER SEVEN

Snacks and Sides

◄ *Vegetable Couscous, page 90*

Cinnamon Apple Chips

SERVES 4 • PREP TIME: 5 MINUTES • COOK TIME: 2 TO 3 HOURS

There's something about crunchy snacks like chips that leave you reaching for more. This guilt-free chip provides vitamins, fiber, and delicious flavor all in one. Cinnamon, an aromatic and warming spice, aides in digestion and supports the spleen, kidneys, and lungs, making it a great addition to your diet and to these chips.

4 apples
1 teaspoon ground
   cinnamon

1 Preheat the oven to 200°F. Line a baking sheet with parchment paper.

2 Core the apples and cut into ⅛-inch slices.

3 In a medium bowl, toss the apple slices with the cinnamon. Spread the apples in a single layer on the prepared baking sheet.

4 Cook for 2 to 3 hours, until the apples are dry. They will still be soft while hot, but will crisp once completely cooled. Store in an airtight container for up to four days.

Cooking tip: If you don't have parchment paper, use cooking spray to prevent sticking.

Per Serving Calories: 96; Total Fat: 0g; Saturated Fat: 0g; Cholesterol: 0mg; Carbohydrates: 26g; Fiber: 5g; Protein: 1g; Phosphorus: 0mg; Potassium: 198mg; Sodium: 2mg

Savory Collard Chips

SERVES 4 • PREP TIME: 5 MINUTES • COOK TIME: 20 MINUTES

If you like kale chips, you'll probably love collard chips. The sturdy green holds up well to baking, creating a crisp chip that is perfect for anytime snacking. The simple mix of herbs adds a garlicky kick to the chips, which will ensure that you are getting plenty of vegetables in your diet—even if they don't feel like vegetables.

1 bunch collard greens

1 teaspoon extra-virgin olive oil

Juice of ½ lemon

½ teaspoon garlic powder

¼ teaspoon freshly ground black pepper

1 Preheat the oven to 350°F. Line a baking sheet with parchment paper.

2 Cut the collards into 2-by-2-inch squares and pat dry with paper towels. In a large bowl, toss the greens with the olive oil, lemon juice, garlic powder, and pepper. Use your hands to mix well, massaging the dressing into the greens until evenly coated.

3 Arrange the collards in a single layer on the baking sheet, and cook for 8 minutes. Flip the pieces and cook for an additional 8 minutes, until crisp. Remove from the oven, let cool, and store in an airtight container in a cool location for up to three days.

Substitution tip: *If you prefer, use fresh garlic instead of dried. Mince 2 or 3 cloves, toss with the collards, and proceed as directed.*

Per Serving Calories: 24; Total Fat: 1g; Saturated Fat: 0g; Cholesterol: 0mg; Carbohydrates: 3g; Fiber: 1g; Protein: 1g; Phosphorus: 6mg; Potassium: 72mg; Sodium: 8mg

Roasted Red Pepper Hummus

SERVES 8 • PREP TIME: 10 MINUTES • COOK TIME: 10 MINUTES

Hummus is generally considered a healthy food, but like many other processed foods, store-bought versions are filled with sodium and preservatives. Make this simple hummus at home to keep sodium levels in check, and keep the serving size to 2 tablespoons. This is easy if you use it as a spread on sandwiches, or make vegetables the star and dip them in hummus for a quick snack.

1 red bell pepper

1 (15-ounce) can chickpeas, drained and rinsed

Juice of 1 lemon

2 tablespoons tahini

2 garlic cloves

2 tablespoons extra-virgin olive oil

1. Move an oven rack to the highest position. Heat the broiler to high.

2. Core the pepper and cut it into three or four large pieces. Arrange them on a baking sheet, skin-side up.

3. Broil the peppers for 5 to 10 minutes, until the skins are charred. Remove from the oven and transfer the peppers to a small bowl. Cover with plastic wrap and let them steam for 10 to 15 minutes, until cool enough to handle.

4. Peel the charred skin off the peppers, and place the peppers in a blender.

5. Add the chickpeas, lemon juice, tahini, garlic, and olive oil. Process until smooth, adding up to 1 tablespoon of water to adjust consistency as desired.

Substitution tip: *This hummus can also be made without the red pepper if desired. To do this, simply follow Step 5. This will cut the potassium to 59mg per serving.*

Per Serving Calories: 103; Total Fat: 6g; Saturated Fat: 1g; Cholesterol: 0mg; Carbohydrates: 10g; Fiber: 3g; Protein: 3g; Phosphorus: 58mg; Potassium: 91mg; Sodium: 72mg

Thai-Style Eggplant Dip

SERVES 4 • PREP TIME: 10 MINUTES • COOK TIME: 30 MINUTES

In hot climates, such as Thailand, eggplant is commonplace as a cooling vegetable with its sweet flavor. Here it's mixed with sweet, savory, and spicy elements to create a fantastic dip that is just right for vegetables or crackers.

1 pound Thai eggplant
  (or Japanese or
  Chinese eggplant)
2 tablespoons rice vinegar
2 teaspoons sugar
1 teaspoon low-sodium
  soy sauce
1 jalapeño pepper
2 garlic cloves
¼ cup chopped basil
Cut vegetables or
  crackers, for serving

1 Preheat the oven to 425°F.

2 Pierce the eggplant in several places with a skewer or knife. Place on a rimmed baking sheet and cook until soft, about 30 minutes. Let cool, cut in half, and scoop out the flesh of the eggplant into a blender.

3 Add the rice vinegar, sugar, soy sauce, jalapeño, garlic, and basil to the blender. Process until smooth. Serve with cut vegetables or crackers.

Lower sodium tip: If you need to lower your sodium further, omit the soy sauce to lower the sodium to 3mg.

Per Serving Calories: 40; Total Fat: 0g; Saturated Fat: 0g; Cholesterol: 0mg; Carbohydrates: 10g; Fiber: 4g; Protein: 2g; Phosphorus: 34mg; Potassium: 284mg; Sodium: 47mg

Collard Salad Rolls with Peanut Dipping Sauce

SERVES 4 • PREP TIME: 20 MINUTES

These delicious Asian-inspired rolls allow you to creatively load up on vegetables. Perfect as a midday snack or light lunch, the rolls possess a wonderful variety of textures and flavor, and when dunked in the sweet-and-spicy peanut-butter dipping sauce, they'll reward you with an explosion of taste.

FOR THE DIPPING SAUCE

¼ cup peanut butter

2 tablespoons honey

Juice of 1 lime

¼ teaspoon red chili flakes

FOR THE SALAD ROLLS

4 ounces extra-firm tofu

1 bunch collard greens

1 cup thinly sliced
   purple cabbage

1 cup bean sprouts

2 carrots,
   cut into matchsticks

½ cup cilantro leaves
   and stems

TO MAKE THE DIPPING SAUCE

In a blender, combine the peanut butter, honey, lime juice, and chili flakes, and process until smooth. Add 1 to 2 tablespoons of water as desired for consistency.

TO MAKE THE SALAD ROLLS

1   Using paper towels, press the excess moisture from the tofu. Cut into ½-inch-thick matchsticks.

2   Remove any tough stems from the collard greens and set aside.

3   Arrange all of the ingredients within reach. Cup one collard green leaf in your hand, and add a couple pieces of the tofu and a small amount each of the cabbage, bean sprouts, and carrots. Top with a couple cilantro sprigs, and roll into a cylinder. Place each roll, seam-side down, on a serving platter while you assemble the rest of the rolls. Serve with the dipping sauce.

Substitution tip: *To lower the potassium, omit the cabbage and use only 1 carrot, which will drop the potassium to 208mg.*

Per Serving Calories: 174; Total Fat: 9g; Saturated Fat: 2g; Cholesterol: 0mg; Carbohydrates: 20g; Fiber: 5g; Protein: 8g; Phosphorus: 56mg; Potassium: 284mg; Sodium: 42mg

Simple Roasted Broccoli

SERVES 6 • PREP TIME: 5 MINUTES • COOK TIME: 20 MINUTES

Roasting is the ideal way to prepare broccoli because it brings out the vegetable's natural sweetness. This simple side is perfect for any weeknight meal and tastes so good you'll likely be inspired to eat the cruciferous powerhouse more often. Broccoli is loaded with twice the vitamin C of an orange, nearly as much calcium as whole milk, and powerful antioxidants and immune-boosting compounds, making it the perfect side to just about any meal.

2 small heads broccoli, cut into florets

1 tablespoon extra-virgin olive oil

3 garlic cloves, minced

1 Preheat the oven to 425°F.

2 In a medium bowl, toss the broccoli with the olive oil and garlic. Arrange in a single layer on a baking sheet.

3 Roast for 10 minutes, then flip the broccoli and roast an additional 10 minutes. Serve.

Cooking tip: *Roasted broccoli makes for great leftovers—throw them in a quick salad for added flavor and bulk. To save leftovers, refrigerate in an airtight container for three to five days.*

Per Serving Calories: 38; Total Fat: 2g; Saturated Fat: 0g; Cholesterol: 0mg; Carbohydrates: 4g; Fiber: 1g; Protein: 1g; Phosphorus: 32mg; Potassium: 150mg; Sodium: 15mg

Roasted Mint Carrots

SERVES 6 • PREP TIME: 5 MINUTES • COOK TIME: 20 MINUTES

Carrots are a great source of the antioxidant vitamin A, and although high in potassium, consumed in moderation carrots can be a healthy part of your diet. In this preparation, roasting enhances the vegetable's natural sweetness while mint adds a complementary flavor. There are several hundred varieties of carrots, but seek out those with the deepest orange color, as they contain the most vitamin A.

1 pound carrots, trimmed

1 tablespoon
   extra-virgin olive oil

Freshly ground
   black pepper

¼ cup thinly sliced mint

1 Preheat the oven to 425°F.

2 Arrange the carrots in a single layer on a rimmed baking sheet. Drizzle with the olive oil, and shake the carrots on the sheet to coat. Season with pepper.

3 Roast for 20 minutes, or until tender and browned, stirring twice while cooking. Sprinkle with the mint and serve.

Substitution tip: *To lower the potassium in this dish, use 8 ounces of carrots and 8 ounces of turnips cut into cubes. This will cut the potassium to 193mg.*

Per Serving Calories: 51; Total Fat: 2g; Saturated Fat: 0g; Cholesterol: 0mg; Carbohydrates: 7g; Fiber: 2g; Protein: 1g; Phosphorus: 26mg; Potassium: 242mg; Sodium: 52mg

Roasted Root Vegetables

SERVES 6 • PREP TIME: 10 MINUTES • COOK TIME: 25 MINUTES

Root vegetables have a comfort-food appeal that makes them great for pairing with meat, fish, and poultry dishes. Turnips, rutabaga, and parsnips may not be the first root vegetables you think of, but these nutritional powerhouses are well worth experimenting with. Roasting accentuates their sweetness, resulting in a tender mix that's loaded with flavor but doesn't overwhelm the main course. Look for young and tender vegetables—you don't need to peel them, so prep time is short.

1 cup chopped turnips

1 cup chopped rutabaga

1 cup chopped parsnips

1 tablespoon
   extra-virgin olive oil

1 teaspoon fresh
   chopped rosemary

Freshly ground
   black pepper

1 Preheat the oven to 400°F.

2 In a large bowl, toss the turnips, rutabaga, and parsnips with the olive oil and rosemary. Arrange in a single layer on a baking sheet, and season with pepper.

3 Bake until the vegetables are tender and browned, 20 to 25 minutes, stirring once.

Substitution tip: *Experiment with other fresh herbs in this dish to suit your own tastes. Thyme, tarragon, oregano, and minced garlic all add unique flavors to these root vegetables.*

Per Serving Calories: 52; Total Fat: 2g; Saturated Fat: 0g; Cholesterol: 0mg; Carbohydrates: 7g; Fiber: 2g; Protein: 1g; Phosphorus: 35mg; Potassium: 205mg; Sodium: 22mg

Vegetable Couscous

SERVES 6 • PREP TIME: 10 MINUTES • COOK TIME: 15 MINUTES

Couscous is a quick-cooking refined grain product, great for weeknight meals. Simply add to boiling water, cover, let stand for just under 10 minutes, and voilà— this delicious grain is ready! Combined with vegetables, this filling side dish pairs well with meat, seafood, and chicken.

1 tablespoon
   extra-virgin olive oil

½ sweet onion, diced

1 carrot, diced

1 celery stalk, diced

½ cup diced red or
   yellow bell pepper

1 small zucchini, diced

1 cup couscous

1½ cups Simple Chicken
   Broth (page 180)
   or low-sodium
   store-bought
   chicken stock

½ teaspoon garlic powder

Freshly ground
   black pepper

1 In a large skillet, heat the olive oil over medium heat. Add the onion, carrot, celery, and bell pepper, and cook, stirring occasionally, until the vegetables are just becoming tender, about 5 to 7 minutes.

2 Add the zucchini, couscous, broth, and garlic powder. Stir to blend, and bring to a boil. Cover and remove from the heat. Let stand for 5 to 8 minutes. Fluff with a fork, season with pepper, and serve.

Substitution tip: *Swap out vegetables to make this couscous your own creation. Yellow summer squash or pattypan squash can be substituted for the zucchini. Other vegetables, like asparagus, broccoli, or cauliflower, can be added instead of carrots and bell peppers.*

Per Serving Calories: 154; Total Fat: 3g; Saturated Fat: 1g; Cholesterol: 0mg; Carbohydrates: 27g; Fiber: 2g; Protein: 5g; Phosphorus: 83mg; Potassium: 197mg; Sodium: 36mg

Garlic Cauliflower Rice

SERVES 8 • PREP TIME: 5 MINUTES • COOK TIME: 10 MINUTES

Cauliflower rice is a clever vegetable-based alternative to white or brown rice. In this version, garlic and freshly ground black pepper make for a flavorful blend that goes well with both meat and vegetarian dishes. Because cauliflower is high in potassium, I recommend keeping the serving size at just ½ cup.

1 medium head cauliflower
1 tablespoon
    extra-virgin olive oil
4 garlic cloves, minced
Freshly ground
    black pepper

1 Using a sharp knife, remove the core of the cauliflower, and separate the cauliflower into florets.

2 In a food processor, pulse the florets until they are the size of rice, being careful not to overprocess them to the point of becoming mushy.

3 In a large skillet over medium heat, heat the olive oil. Add the garlic, and stir until just fragrant.

4 Add the cauliflower, stirring to coat. Add 1 tablespoon of water to the pan, cover, and reduce the heat to low. Steam for 7 to 10 minutes, until the cauliflower is tender. Season with pepper and serve.

Cooking tip: Cauliflower rice tastes great both when fresh and after resting in the refrigerator for a day or two. Make a batch and use it throughout the week as a side dish, heating it in the microwave before serving. In an airtight container, it will keep refrigerated for three to five days.

Per Serving Calories: 37; Total Fat: 2g; Saturated Fat: 0g; Cholesterol: 0mg; Carbohydrates: 4g; Fiber: 2g; Protein: 2g; Phosphorus: 35mg; Potassium: 226mg; Sodium: 22mg

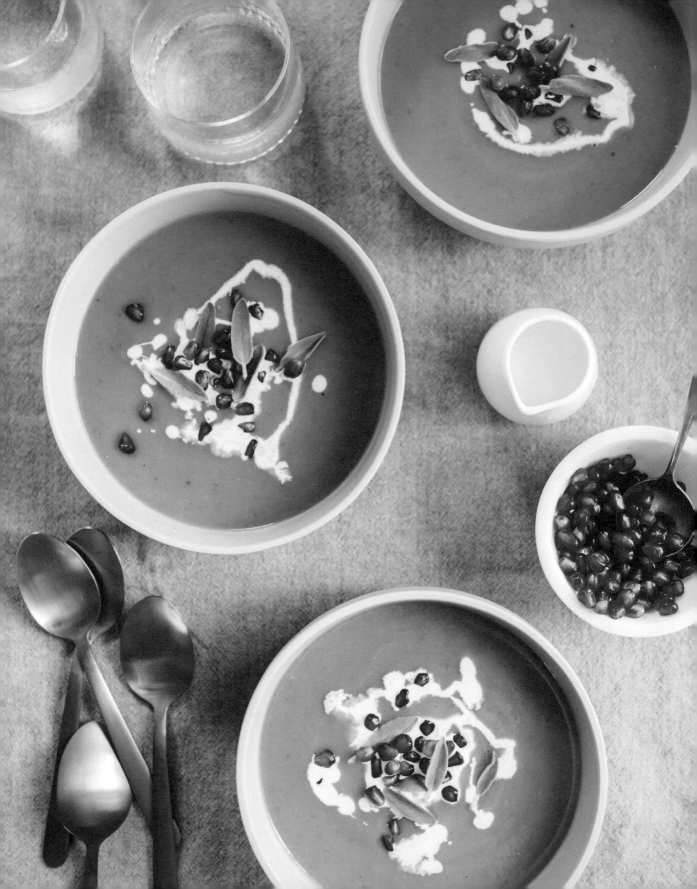

Soups

◄ *Golden Beet Soup, page 96*

Creamy Broccoli Soup

SERVES 4 • PREP TIME: 10 MINUTES • COOK TIME: 15 MINUTES

Creamy broccoli soup is equal parts simple and delicious. Most broccoli soups get their creaminess from whole milk, cream, or cheese—but this recipe cleverly creates the same consistency using lower-fat rice milk and a bit of Parmesan. With intense fresh flavor and richness, this superb weekday soup tastes even better after a couple days' rest in the refrigerator.

1 teaspoon extra-virgin
   olive oil

½ sweet onion,
   roughly chopped

2 cups chopped broccoli

4 cups low-sodium
   vegetable broth

Freshly ground
   black pepper

1 cup Homemade
   Rice Milk (page 70)
   or unsweetened
   store-bought rice milk

¼ cup grated
   Parmesan cheese

1 In a medium saucepan over medium-high heat, heat the olive oil. Add the onion and cook for 3 to 5 minutes, until it begins to soften. Add the broccoli and broth, and season with pepper.

2 Bring to a boil, reduce the heat, and simmer uncovered for 10 minutes, until the broccoli is just tender but still bright green.

3 Transfer the soup mixture to a blender. Add the rice milk, and process until smooth. Return to the saucepan, stir in the Parmesan cheese, and serve.

Substitution tip: *You can use this recipe to make several varieties of green soups. Experiment substituting spinach, a mix of arugula and kale, or microgreens, for a twist on the ordinary that suits your tastes.*

Per Serving Calories: 88; Total Fat: 3g; Saturated Fat: 1g; Cholesterol: 6mg; Carbohydrates: 12g; Fiber: 3g; Protein: 4g; Phosphorus: 87mg; Potassium: 201mg; Sodium: 281mg

Curried Carrot and Beet Soup

SERVES 4 • PREP TIME: 10 MINUTES • COOK TIME: 50 MINUTES

This vibrantly colored carrot and beet soup is loaded with vitamins and flavor. The anti-inflammatory beets help support the kidneys, and the carrots are a great source of beta-carotene. Curry powder ties the flavors together, and a generous portion of rice milk makes the soup creamy and satiating.

1 large red beet

5 carrots, chopped

1 tablespoon curry powder

3 cups Homemade
   Rice Milk (page 70)
   or unsweetened
   store-bought rice milk

Freshly ground
   black pepper

Yogurt, for serving

1. Preheat the oven to 400°F.

2. Wrap the beet in aluminum foil and roast for 45 minutes, until the vegetable is tender when pierced with a fork. Remove from the oven and let cool.

3. In a saucepan, add the carrots and cover with water. Bring to a boil, reduce the heat, cover, and simmer for 10 minutes, until tender.

4. Transfer the carrots and beet to a food processor, and process until smooth. Add the curry powder and rice milk. Season with pepper. Serve topped with a dollop of yogurt.

Substitution tip: *Carrots are high in potassium. If you need to reduce your potassium further, use 2 carrots instead of 5. The soup will be a little thinner but still have a carrot flavor and just 322mg of potassium.*

Per Serving Calories: 112; Total Fat: 1g; Saturated Fat: 0g; Cholesterol: 0mg; Carbohydrates: 24g; Fiber: 7g; Protein: 3g; Phosphorus: 57mg; Potassium: 468mg; Sodium: 129mg

Golden Beet Soup

SERVES 4 • PREP TIME: 10 MINUTES • COOK TIME: 35 MINUTES

Golden beets taste the same as red beets but lack the red-pigment betalain, which gives way to this eye-catching golden soup. The trio of pomegranate seeds, sage, and crème fraîche adds additional bright color along with a satisfying crunch and savory goodness. As with any hot soup, purée with caution and fill the blender only to the recommended level to prevent splattering the hot soup.

3 tablespoons
  unsalted butter

4 golden beets, cut
  into ½-inch cubes

½ sweet onion, chopped

1-inch piece ginger, minced

Zest and juice of 1 lemon

4 cups Simple Chicken
  Broth (page 180)
  or low-sodium
  store-bought
  chicken stock

Freshly ground
  black pepper

¼ cup pomegranate
  seeds, for serving

¼ cup crème fraîche,
  for serving (see
  Substitution tip)

10 sage leaves, for serving

1 In a medium saucepan over medium heat, melt the butter.

2 Add the beets, onion, ginger, and lemon zest, and cover. Cook, stirring occasionally, for 15 minutes. Add the broth, and continue to cook for 20 more minutes, until the beets are very tender.

3 In batches, transfer the soup to a blender and purée, or use an immersion blender.

4 Return the soup to the saucepan, and season with the pepper and lemon juice.

5 Serve topped with the pomegranate seeds, crème fraîche, and sage leaves.

Substitution tip: *You can buy crème fraîche at many grocery stores, or make your own. If you don't have crème fraîche, a dollop of whole-milk yogurt is a fine substitute.*

Per Serving Calories: 186; Total Fat: 11g; Saturated Fat: 7g; Cholesterol: 26mg; Carbohydrates: 17g; Fiber: 3g; Protein: 7g; Phosphorus: 125mg; Potassium: 557mg; Sodium: 148mg

Asparagus Lemon Soup

SERVES 4 • PREP TIME: 10 MINUTES • COOK TIME: 25 MINUTES

Asparagus soup can become dull and muted when overcooked, but this creamy soup is brightened fantastically with the addition of lemon. Trim the asparagus tips and set them aside to add at the end of cooking, as a tender accompaniment that enriches texture, flavor, and color.

1 pound asparagus

2 tablespoons extra-virgin olive oil

½ sweet onion, chopped

4 cups low-sodium chicken stock

½ cup Homemade Rice Milk (page 70) or unsweetened store-bought rice milk

Freshly ground black pepper

Juice of 1 lemon

1 Cut the asparagus tips from the spears and set aside.

2 In a small stockpot over medium heat, heat the olive oil. Add the onion and cook, stirring frequently for 3 to 5 minutes, until it begins to soften.

3 Add the stock and asparagus stalks, and bring to a boil. Reduce the heat and simmer until the asparagus is tender, about 15 minutes.

4 Transfer to a blender or food processor, and carefully purée until smooth. Return to the pot, add the asparagus tips, and simmer until tender, about 5 minutes.

5 Add the rice milk, pepper, and lemon juice, and stir until heated through. Serve.

Cooking tip: Make this soup up to three days in advance and store in the refrigerator. When ready to serve, heat in the microwave or on the stove top.

Per Serving Calories: 145; Total Fat: 9g; Saturated Fat: 1g; Cholesterol: 0mg; Carbohydrates: 13g; Fiber: 3g; Protein: 8g; Phosphorus: 143mg; Potassium: 497mg; Sodium: 92mg

Cauliflower and Chive Soup

SERVES 4 • PREP TIME: 10 MINUTES • COOK TIME: 20 MINUTES

Cauliflower is a terrific vegetable for a savory soup. Wonderfully creamy, it has a mild flavor that can be easily manipulated to suit your tastes. A full head of cauliflower forms the backbone of the soup, topped off with a generous sprinkling of chives, to create a flavorful and satisfying lunch.

2 tablespoons
   extra-virgin olive oil
½ sweet onion, chopped
2 garlic cloves, minced
2 cups Simple Chicken
   Broth (page 180)
   or low-sodium
   store-bought
   chicken stock
1 cauliflower head,
   broken into florets
Freshly ground
   black pepper
4 tablespoons (¼ cup)
   finely chopped chives

1 In a small stockpot over medium heat, heat the olive oil. Add the onion and cook, stirring frequently, for 3 to 5 minutes, until it begins to soften. Add the garlic and stir until fragrant.

2 Add the broth and cauliflower, and bring to a boil. Reduce the heat and simmer until the cauliflower is tender, about 15 minutes.

3 Transfer the soup in batches to a blender or food processor and purée until smooth, or use an immersion blender. Return the soup to the pot, and season with pepper. Before serving, top each bowl with 1 tablespoon of chives.

Cooking tip: If you're using a traditional blender, work in batches, and place a clean kitchen towel over the top of the lid as you blend to prevent splashing hot soup. Fill the blender only to the safe-fill line, and be very cautious as you go, as hot liquids can be dangerous to work with.

Per Serving Calories: 132; Total Fat: 8g; Saturated Fat: 1g; Cholesterol: 0mg; Carbohydrates: 13g; Fiber: 3g; Protein: 6g; Phosphorus: 116mg; Potassium: 607mg; Sodium: 84mg

Bulgur and Greens Soup with Soft-Boiled Egg

SERVES 4 • PREP TIME: 10 MINUTES • COOK TIME: 20 MINUTES

The star of this soup? The mustard greens—the most pungent variety of greens from the cabbage family. However, when it's cooked in broth, like here, the flavorful greens become significantly milder and create a wonderful contrast to the neutral-flavored bulgur. A soft-boiled egg ties the soup together—enjoy watching the runny yolk mix into the broth as you devour the bowl.

1 cup bulgur

4 eggs

4 cups Simple Chicken
   Broth (page 180)
   or low-sodium
   store-bought
   chicken stock

1 bunch mustard greens,
   thick stems removed,
   coarsely chopped

Freshly ground
   black pepper

2 scallions, thinly sliced

2-inch piece ginger,
   julienned

2 celery stalks, thinly sliced

1 In a small pot, add the bulgur to 2 cups of water and bring to a boil. Cover, reduce the heat, and simmer for 10 to 15 minutes, until the bulgur is tender. Drain the bulgur and set aside.

2 Place the whole eggs in a small bowl. Bring a pot of water to a boil, and carefully pour the water over the eggs. Let sit for 8 minutes, or longer if a more-set egg is desired. Carefully peel the eggs and set aside.

3 In a medium stockpot, bring the broth to a simmer. Add the mustard greens, season with pepper, and cook until tender, 3 to 5 minutes.

4 Divide the bulgur between four bowls, and add 1 cup of broth to each bowl. Divide the mustard greens between the bowls. Add 1 egg to each bowl. Top with the scallions, ginger, and celery. Serve.

Substitution tip: *If you can't find mustard greens, feel free to substitute any other type of green. Turnip greens, collard greens, or spinach all work well. If you are using a green with thick stems, like turnip or collard greens, remove the stems before cooking.*

Per Serving Calories: 257; Total Fat: 7g; Saturated Fat: 2g; Cholesterol: 208mg; Carbohydrates: 34g; Fiber: 8g; Protein: 18g; Phosphorus: 315mg; Potassium: 661mg; Sodium: 186mg

Vegetable Lentil Soup

SERVES 4 • PREP TIME: 10 MINUTES • COOK TIME: 25 MINUTES

Lentil soup tops the charts as a cool-weather soup, and this hearty version will not disappoint. Carrots, celery, and chard round out this colorful classic, and a splash of lemon at the end of cooking boosts flavor and brightness.

1 tablespoon
    extra-virgin olive oil

½ sweet onion, diced

2 carrots, diced

2 celery stalks, diced

½ cup lentils

5 cups Simple Chicken
    Broth (page 180)
    or low-sodium
    store-bought
    chicken stock

2 cups sliced
    chard leaves

Freshly ground
    black pepper

Juice of 1 lemon

1   In a medium stockpot over medium-high heat, heat the olive oil. Add the onion and stir until softened, about 3 to 5 minutes.

2   Add the carrots, celery, lentils, and broth. Bring to a boil, reduce the heat and simmer, uncovered, for 15 minutes, until the lentils are tender.

3   Add the chard and cook for 3 additional minutes, until wilted.

4   Season with the pepper and lemon juice. Serve.

Substitution tip: You can use any greens that you have on hand for this soup; just adjust cooking times as needed based on the type. Collard, mustard, and turnip greens will need more cooking time, while spinach or bok choy will require just a couple minutes, much like chard.

Per Serving Calories: 195; Total Fat: 6g; Saturated Fat: 1g; Cholesterol: 0mg; Carbohydrates: 25g; Fiber: 9g; Protein: 13g; Phosphorus: 228mg; Potassium: 707mg; Sodium: 157mg

Simple Chicken and Rice Soup

SERVES 4 • PREP TIME: 10 MINUTES • COOK TIME: 15 MINUTES

Chicken soup exemplifies classic comfort food, and this one's easy to throw together in a pinch. It starts with raw chicken, but you can cut out a step by starting with already-cooked chopped or shredded chicken. Either way, be sure not to skip the thyme, which adds a characteristic and inviting aroma to the soup without overpowering the other flavors.

1 tablespoon
    extra-virgin olive oil

½ sweet onion, chopped

2 celery stalks, chopped

2 carrots, chopped

8 ounces chicken
    breast, diced

4 cups Simple Chicken
    Broth (page 180)
    or low-sodium
    store-bought
    chicken stock

¼ teaspoon dried
    thyme leaves

1 cup cooked rice

Juice of 1 lime

Freshly ground
    black pepper

2 tablespoons chopped
    parsley leaves,
    for garnish

1 In a medium stockpot, heat the olive oil over medium-high heat. Add the onion, celery, and carrots, and cook, stirring often, for about 5 minutes, until the onion begins to soften.

2 Add the chicken breast and continue stirring until the meat is just browned but not cooked through. Add the broth and thyme, and bring to a boil. Reduce the heat and simmer for 10 minutes, until the chicken is cooked through and the vegetables are tender.

3 Add the rice and lime juice. Season with pepper. Serve, garnished with parsley leaves.

Lower sodium tip: Choosing the Simple Chicken Broth (page 180) over the store-bought variety will allow you to better control the amount of sodium in the finished product.

Per Serving Calories: 175; Total Fat: 6g; Saturated Fat: 1g; Cholesterol: 33mg; Carbohydrates: 19g; Fiber: 3g; Protein: 13g; Phosphorus: 217mg; Potassium: 403mg; Sodium: 227mg

Chicken Pho

SERVES 4 • PREP TIME: 10 MINUTES • COOK TIME: 15 MINUTES

Pho is a popular Vietnamese noodle soup, characterized by rice noodles, broth, a variety of herbs, and meat. Traditional phos are long-simmered to create the perfect broth, but in this version, low-sodium chicken broth makes for a quick soup without fuss. Served with a medley of basil, bean sprouts, jalapeño, scallions, and cilantro, the freshness of this soup really shines through.

5 cups Simple Chicken
    Broth (page 180)
    or low-sodium
    store-bought
    chicken stock
1-inch piece ginger,
    cut lengthwise into
    2 or 3 strips
1 cup cooked chicken
    breast, diced
Several fresh Thai
    basil sprigs
1 cup mung bean sprouts
1 lime, cut into wedges
1 jalapeño pepper,
    stemmed, seeded,
    and thinly sliced
1 (16-ounce) package dried
    rice vermicelli noodles,
    cooked according to
    package directions
4 tablespoons (¼ cup)
    sliced scallions
4 tablespoons (¼ cup)
    chopped cilantro leaves

1 In a medium stockpot over medium-high heat, add the broth and ginger, and bring to a simmer. Add the chicken and simmer for 5 minutes. Remove the ginger from the pot and discard.

2 On a plate, arrange the Thai basil, bean sprouts, lime wedges, and jalapeño slices.

3 Distribute the noodles among four bowls. Add 1¼ cups of broth to each bowl. Top with 1 tablespoon each of the scallions and cilantro. Serve immediately, alongside the plate of garnishes.

Substitution tip: If you can't find fresh Thai basil near you, you can substitute regular basil, available in the fresh herb section of your grocery store.

Per Serving Calories: 325; Total Fat: 3g; Saturated Fat: 1g; Cholesterol: 30mg; Carbohydrates: 55g; Fiber: 2g; Protein: 21g; Phosphorus: 205mg; Potassium: 389mg; Sodium: 313mg

Turkey Burger Soup

SERVES 4 • PREP TIME: 10 MINUTES • COOK TIME: 25 MINUTES

You'll feel like you are eating a burger in a bowl with this hearty soup that makes a filling lunch or dinner. To keep sodium levels low, be sure to drain the liquids from the tomatoes before adding them to the pot. The combination of basil, oregano, and thyme creates a flavorful trio that the whole family will enjoy.

2 tablespoons extra-virgin olive oil

1 pound ground turkey breast

½ sweet onion, chopped

3 garlic cloves, minced

Freshly ground black pepper

1 (16-ounce) can low-sodium diced tomatoes, drained

4 cups Simple Chicken Broth (page 180) or low-sodium store-bought chicken stock

1 cup sliced carrots

1 cup sliced celery

1 tablespoon chopped fresh basil

1 tablespoon chopped fresh oregano

1 tablespoon chopped fresh thyme

1. In a medium stockpot over medium-high heat, heat the olive oil. Add the turkey, onion, and garlic, and cook, stirring frequently, until the turkey is browned. Season with pepper.

2. Add the drained tomatoes, broth, carrots, celery, basil, oregano, and thyme. Reduce the heat to low, and simmer for 20 minutes. Serve.

Substitution tip: *If you don't have fresh basil, oregano, or thyme, use dried instead. Substitute 1 teaspoon of dried herbs for each tablespoon of fresh.*

Per Serving Calories: 260; Total Fat: 9g; Saturated Fat: 1g; Cholesterol: 282mg; Carbohydrates: 19g; Fiber: 4g; Protein: 29g; Phosphorus: 106mg; Potassium: 449mg; Sodium: 296mg

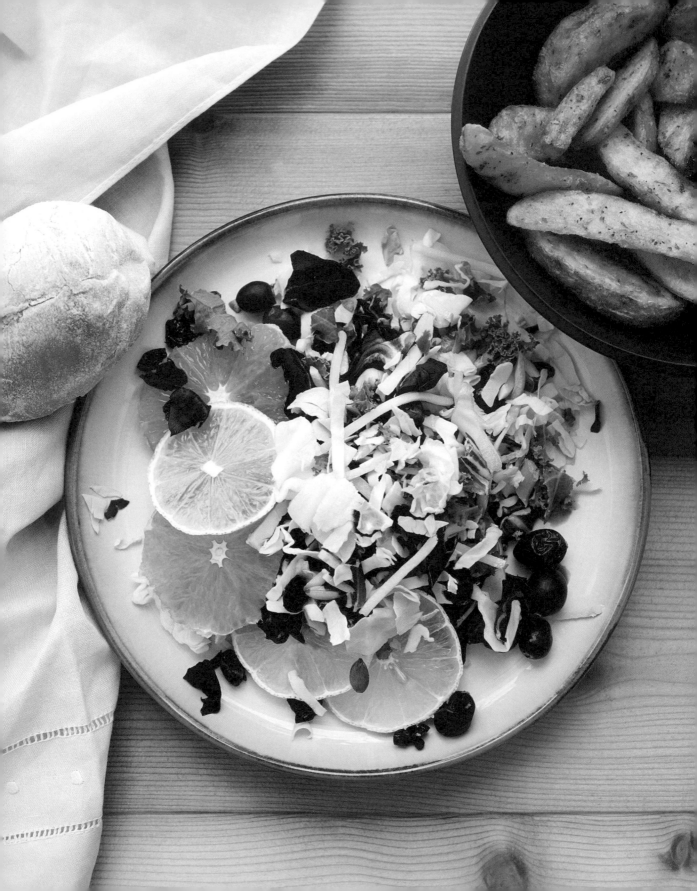

Salads

◄ *Mixed Green Leaf and Citrus Salad, page 109*

Celery and Arugula Salad

SERVES 4 • PREP TIME: 10 MINUTES

Peppery arugula makes a wonderful complement to the crunch of celery in this salad. Arugula is a bitter digestive aide and a terrific source of vitamins A and C, calcium, and folic acid. Find it in markets in the spring, early summer, and fall, or try your hand at growing your own. Arugula is easy to grow from seeds and will provide you with plenty of salads in no time.

1 shallot, thinly sliced

3 celery stalks, cut into 1-inch pieces about ¼ inch thick

2 cups loosely packed arugula

1 tablespoon extra-virgin olive oil

2 tablespoons white wine vinegar

Freshly ground black pepper

2 tablespoons grated Parmesan cheese

1 In a medium bowl, toss the shallot, celery stalks, and arugula.

2 In a small bowl, whisk the olive oil, vinegar, and pepper. Pour the dressing over the salad, and toss to coat. Top with Parmesan cheese and serve.

Substitution tip: *For a milder salad, you can substitute an equal amount of baby salad greens, or mix 1 cup of salad greens and 1 cup of arugula.*

Per Serving Calories: 45; Total Fat: 4g; Saturated Fat: 1g; Cholesterol: 2mg; Carbohydrates: 1g; Fiber: 0g; Protein: 1g; Phosphorus: 23mg; Potassium: 47mg; Sodium: 47mg

Cucumber and Radish Salad

SERVES 6 • PREP TIME: 10 MINUTES

If you love the snap of cucumbers and radishes, this salad will please your palate. Both vegetables are sources of potassium, however, so it's important to keep the serving size to ½ cup. For the best flavor and nutrition, use raw apple cider vinegar, characterized by a cloudy sediment at the bottom of the bottle.

2 large cucumbers, peeled and sliced

1 bunch radishes, sliced

½ sweet onion, sliced

¼ cup apple cider vinegar

1 tablespoon extra-virgin olive oil

Freshly ground black pepper

1 In a medium bowl, toss the cucumbers, radishes, and onion.

2 Add the apple cider vinegar and olive oil, and toss to coat. Season with pepper.

Cooking tip: Make this salad up to two days in advance and store refrigerated in an airtight container until ready for use.

Per Serving Calories: 69; Total Fat: 4g; Saturated Fat: 1g; Cholesterol: 0mg; Carbohydrates: 8g; Fiber: 2g; Protein: 2g; Phosphorus: 52mg; Potassium: 386mg; Sodium: 29mg

Spinach Salad with Orange Vinaigrette

SERVES 4 • PREP TIME: 5 MINUTES

This super-quick, refreshing salad presents itself with a touch of sweetness and a treasure trove of nutrients. Vitamins A, C, K, and fiber are just a few of its hidden health benefits. To ensure that the greens stay crispy, toss the salad with the vinaigrette right before serving.

Zest and juice of
   1 mandarin orange
1 tablespoon
   extra-virgin olive oil
Freshly ground
   black pepper
6 ounces baby spinach
2 mandarin oranges,
   peeled, membranes
   removed

1 In a small bowl, whisk the orange zest, orange juice, and olive oil. Season with pepper.

2 In a medium bowl, toss the spinach and pieces of orange. Drizzle the dressing over the salad, and toss to coat. Serve.

Substitution tip: *To make this a heartier salad that can stand alone as a meal, add 1 cup of diced avocado. This will increase the fat content to 9g, the phosphorus to 53mg, and the potassium to 535mg.*

Per Serving Calories: 73; Total Fat: 4g; Saturated Fat: 1g; Cholesterol: 0mg; Carbohydrates: 10g; Fiber: 2g; Protein: 2g; Phosphorus: 33mg; Potassium: 353mg; Sodium: 35mg

Mixed Green Leaf and Citrus Salad

SERVES 4 • PREP TIME: 10 MINUTES

This sweet and savory combination of citrus, olives, and cranberries is nothing short of addictive. Pepitas, which are hulled pumpkin seeds of a South and Central American variety of squash, contain more protein than many other nuts and seeds, plus they provide the salad with a great crunch. Used sparingly here because of that protein, the pepitas combine with cranberries and olives to create a fun mix of textures and flavors.

4 cups mixed salad greens

¼ cup pepitas

Juice of 1 lemon

2 teaspoons
extra-virgin olive oil

Freshly ground
black pepper

1 orange, peeled and
thinly sliced

½ lemon, peeled and
thinly sliced

4 tablespoons (¼ cup)
dried cranberries

4 tablespoons (¼ cup)
pitted Kalamata olives

1 In a large bowl, toss the greens, pepitas, lemon juice, and olive oil. Season with pepper.

2 Arrange the greens on four plates, and top each with 2 slices of orange and lemon. Add 1 tablespoon each of cranberries and Kalamata olives to each plate. Serve.

Ingredient tip: Toasted pepitas are delicious in this salad. To toast them, preheat the oven to 325°F. Toss the pepitas with ½ teaspoon of olive oil, then spread them on a baking sheet. Roast for about 15 minutes, until golden. Let cool before adding to the salad.

Substitution tip: Use any combination of citrus in this salad for different effects. Sliced grapefruit, limes, and different types of oranges can all be used based on your preference.

Per Serving Calories: 142; Total Fat: 9g; Saturated Fat: 1g; Cholesterol: 0mg; Carbohydrates: 15g; Fiber: 2g; Protein: 3g; Phosphorus: 116mg; Potassium: 219mg; Sodium: 137mg

Roasted Beet Salad

SERVES 4 • PREP TIME: 10 MINUTES • COOK TIME: 30 MINUTES

Roasting vegetables transforms them into sweet morsels, and considering how sweet the beet starts off, its flavor is all the more pronounced when roasted. For a light meal, serve this decadent salad topped with feta and walnuts, or pair it with a poultry or meat dish for something heartier. Select small beets when making this salad—they cook quicker and make for a lovely presentation on the plate.

8 small beets, trimmed

2 tablespoons plus
   1 teaspoon extra-virgin
   olive oil, divided

1 tablespoon white
   wine vinegar

1 teaspoon Dijon mustard

Freshly ground
   black pepper

4 cups baby salad greens

½ sweet onion, sliced

2 tablespoons crumbled
   feta cheese

2 tablespoons
   walnut pieces

1 Preheat the oven to 400°F.

2 Toss the beets with 1 teaspoon of olive oil, wrap them in aluminum foil, and cook for 30 minutes, until fork-tender.

3 In a small bowl, whisk the remaining 2 tablespoons of olive oil, vinegar, and mustard. Season with pepper.

4 In a medium bowl, mix the salad greens, onion, feta cheese, and walnuts. Toss with about half of the vinaigrette. Arrange on four plates.

5 Slice the beets into wedges and top the salads. Serve with the remaining dressing.

Cooking tip: To make this salad in advance, just assemble the salad greens, onion, feta, and walnuts in a bowl—hold off on tossing it with the vinaigrette until ready to serve, to prevent wilting. Store refrigerated up to three days before serving.

Per Serving Calories: 170; Total Fat: 9g; Saturated Fat: 2g; Cholesterol: 4mg; Carbohydrates: 20g; Fiber: 5g; Protein: 4g; Phosphorus: 93mg; Potassium: 585mg; Sodium: 217mg

Pear and Watercress Salad

SERVES 4 • PREP TIME: 10 MINUTES

A pungent herb with a mustard-like flavor, watercress feels surprisingly cool in the mouth. Mixed with pear, this refreshing fall salad simply pops with flavor. For best results, use pears that hold their shape, such as Seckel, Comice, or Bosc.

¼ cup sweet onion, coarsely chopped

1 teaspoon Dijon mustard

2 tablespoons extra-virgin olive oil

1 tablespoon white wine vinegar

1 teaspoon honey

1 bunch watercress, thick stems removed, washed well

2 ripe pears, cored and cut into wedges

1 ounce crumbled feta cheese

1   In a food processor or blender, combine the onion, mustard, olive oil, vinegar, and honey. Process until smooth.

2   In a medium bowl, toss the watercress with the dressing. Arrange on four plates. Top each with pear slices and crumbled feta cheese.

Ingredient tip: Watercress is extremely perishable, so you'll want to buy it within a day or two of using. To store it, place the stems in water without immersing the leaves. When ready to use, wash the leaves in a bowl of water, changing the water out several times before draining and using.

Per Serving Calories: 144; Total Fat: 8g; Saturated Fat: 2g; Cholesterol: 6mg; Carbohydrates: 17g; Fiber: 3g; Protein: 3g; Phosphorus: 70mg; Potassium: 310mg; Sodium: 134mg

Red Coleslaw with Apple

SERVES 4 · PREP TIME: 10 MINUTES

Loaded with anticarcinogenic, antibacterial, antiviral, and antioxidant properties, cabbage is a powerhouse vegetable, and is terrific served raw. In this coleslaw, the red-cabbage variety (which is especially rich in antioxidants) pairs with a tart apple for a unique combination. Serve this salad alongside poultry, pork, or fish.

3 cups shredded
   red cabbage

½ cup shredded carrots

¼ cup finely
   chopped scallions

Juice of 2 lemons

1 tablespoon honey

1 tablespoon
   extra-virgin olive oil

1 large tart apple, peeled
   and finely diced

Freshly ground
   black pepper

In a large bowl, add the cabbage, carrots, scallions, lemon juice, honey, olive oil, and apple. Mix well and refrigerate for 30 minutes to chill. Toss with black pepper right before serving.

Ingredient tip: Cabbage is sold in both red and green varieties. For this recipe, you will need less than a full head of cabbage, so if your store sells halved and wrapped cabbage, you can purchase this to avoid waste. Alternatively, you can save time by buying preshredded cabbage.

Per Serving Calories: 94; Total Fat: 4g; Saturated Fat: 1g; Cholesterol: 0mg; Carbohydrates: 16g; Fiber: 3g; Protein: 2g; Phosphorus: 28mg; Potassium: 303mg; Sodium: 281mg

Roasted Cauliflower with Mixed Greens Salad

SERVES 4 • PREP TIME: 10 MINUTES • COOK TIME: 35 MINUTES

Mixed baby salad greens are ready for anything you throw at them. These mildly flavored greens shine in this simple salad, with just one other vegetable—cauliflower—competing for attention. Roasted until golden brown, the tender cauliflower florets are greeted with a light vinaigrette and a sprinkling of walnut pieces for added texture and protein in this lovely dinner accompaniment.

1 small head cauliflower, cut into small florets

2 tablespoons extra-virgin olive oil, divided

Freshly ground black pepper

6 ounces mixed baby salad greens

2 tablespoons walnut pieces

1 tablespoon apple cider vinegar

1 Preheat the oven to 400°F.

2 In a large bowl, toss the cauliflower with 1 tablespoon of olive oil. Season with pepper. Arrange in a single layer on a large baking sheet.

3 Cook for 30 to 35 minutes, stirring once or twice, until tender and golden brown. Let cool for about 10 minutes.

4 Meanwhile, in a small bowl, mix the remaining tablespoon of olive oil and the vinegar.

5 In a large bowl, toss the mixed salad greens, walnuts, and cauliflower. Just before serving, stir in the olive-oil-and-vinegar mixture, and season with pepper.

Cooking tip: *Make some extra roasted cauliflower as a side, and keep some on hand to whip up this salad without the wait when you need it. It will keep in an airtight container in the refrigerator for three to five days.*

Per Serving Calories: 108; Total Fat: 9g; Saturated Fat: 1g; Cholesterol: 0mg; Carbohydrates: 5g; Fiber: 2g; Protein: 2g; Phosphorus: 42mg; Potassium: 217mg; Sodium: 50mg

Bulgur and Broccoli Salad

SERVES 4 • PREP TIME: 10 MINUTES • COOK TIME: 15 MINUTES

Mint may play a supporting role here, but this cooling herb adds immeasurable brightness to anything it touches. Here the mint is combined with lemon, broccoli, and cherry tomatoes to create a vibrantly flavored salad with the nutty-tasting bulgur at its base. Serve this salad on its own, or spoon it into large lettuce leaves to create a tasty hands-on salad wrap.

3 cups broccoli florets

1 cup bulgur

½ cup cherry
   tomatoes, halved

¼ cup raw sunflower seeds

¼ cup chopped mint leaves

Juice of 1 lemon

1 tablespoon
   extra-virgin olive oil

1 In a medium bowl, prepare an ice-water bath by filling the bowl with ice and water.

2 Fill a medium pot halfway with water and bring to a boil. Add the broccoli and blanch for 3 minutes. With a slotted spoon, remove the broccoli and transfer it to the ice bath, retaining the cooking water over the heat. Once cool, after about 3 minutes, drain the ice and water. Set the broccoli aside.

3 Add the bulgur to the hot water, remove from the heat, cover, and let sit for 15 minutes. Drain, pressing the bulgur with the back of a spoon to remove excess moisture.

4 In a medium bowl, toss the broccoli, bulgur, tomatoes, sunflower seeds, mint, lemon juice, and olive oil. Serve immediately.

Ingredient tip: Bulgur can go rancid quickly, so buy only what you will use in the near future. If possible, smell it for freshness before purchasing, and store it in the refrigerator.

Per Serving Calories: 156; Total Fat: 6g; Saturated Fat: 1g; Cholesterol: 0mg; Carbohydrates: 24g; Fiber: 7g; Protein: 6g; Phosphorus: 101mg; Potassium: 315mg; Sodium: 21mg

Summer Pasta Salad with White Wine Vinaigrette

SERVES 8 • PREP TIME: 10 MINUTES • COOK TIME: 15 MINUTES

Pasta salad is easily transportable and stores well, making it a great component of any meal schedule. Prepare the salad early in the week for quick lunches or serve it alongside dinner. Either way, it holds up well to three or four days of storage in an airtight container. Arugula and garlic give this salad a spicy kick, while the simple white wine vinaigrette enlivens the flavors.

1 pound small pasta
noodles (such as penne,
farfalle, elbow, or rotini)

1 large cucumber, cut
lengthwise and sliced
into half moons

2 cups arugula,
coarsely chopped

3 garlic cloves, minced

2 tablespoons
extra-virgin olive oil

1 tablespoon white
wine vinegar

Freshly ground
black pepper

¼ cup grated
Parmesan cheese

1 Fill a large stockpot halfway with water, and bring to a boil. Add the pasta and cook until al dente. Drain and run the pasta under cold water to stop the cooking.

2 In a large bowl, toss the noodles, cucumber, arugula, and garlic. Drizzle the olive oil and vinegar over the salad, and season with pepper. Stir in the Parmesan cheese and serve.

Substitution tip: *You can use any number of salad greens in this salad. Baby spinach greens, romaine lettuce, and red- and green-leaf lettuces all swap in nicely.*

Per Serving Calories: 227; Total Fat: 4g; Saturated Fat: 1g; Cholesterol: 3mg; Carbohydrates: 43g; Fiber: 5g; Protein: 9g; Phosphorus: 36mg; Potassium: 82mg; Sodium: 60mg

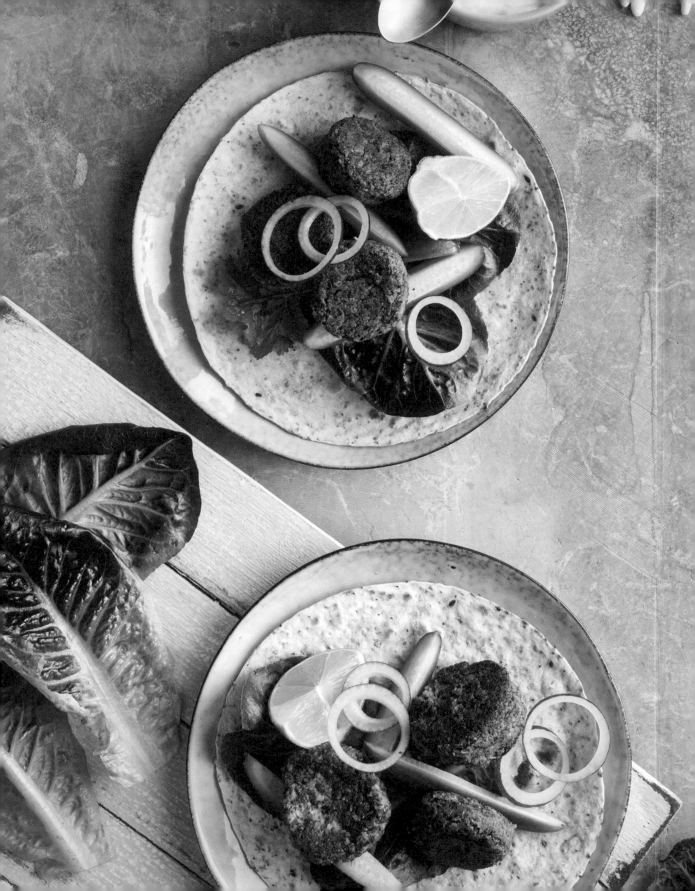

Vegetable Mains

◀ *Spinach Falafel Wrap, page 120*

Cauliflower and Potato Curry

SERVES 4 • PREP TIME: 10 MINUTES • COOK TIME: 15 MINUTES

This classic Indian curry is a lot easier to make at home than you might imagine. Using cauliflower, a potato, and tomatoes, this simple dish comes together in a matter of minutes, and tastes like it demanded a lot more effort. You won't miss the table salt here, because the dish is loaded with aromatic ginger, turmeric, cumin, and garam masala (see Ingredient tip). Serve this curry with rice or flatbread for a satisfying meal.

2 tablespoons canola oil

½ sweet onion, chopped

2-inch piece ginger

3 garlic cloves, minced

1 teaspoon
    ground turmeric

1 teaspoon ground cumin

1 small head cauliflower,
    cut into florets

1 medium potato, diced

2 small tomatoes, diced

1 small green chile,
    stemmed, seeded,
    and diced

½ cup water

Juice of ½ lemon

¼ cup chopped
    cilantro leaves

1 teaspoon garam masala

Rice or bread, for serving

1 In a large pot over medium heat, heat the olive oil. Add the onion and cook, stirring, until softened.

2 Add the ginger and garlic, and cook until fragrant. Stir in the turmeric and cumin. Add the cauliflower, potato, tomatoes, chile, and water. Bring to a simmer, reduce the heat, and cover. Cook, stirring occasionally, for 25 minutes, until the potatoes and cauliflower are tender.

3 Stir in the lemon juice, cilantro, and garam masala. Serve over rice or with bread.

Ingredient tip: Garam masala is a spice blend made up of cumin, coriander, cardamom, black pepper, cinnamon, cloves, nutmeg, and other spices—there are countless variations of the mix. Garam masala is typically added with other spices to curries and South Asian dishes to enhance flavor. Because salt is not added to the blend, a store-bought version is fine, or you can mix your own.

Per Serving Calories: 146; Total Fat: 7g; Saturated Fat: 1g; Cholesterol: 0mg; Carbohydrates: 19g; Fiber: 3g; Protein: 3g; Phosphorus: 65mg; Potassium: 546mg; Sodium: 20mg

White Bean Veggie Burgers

SERVES 4 • PREP TIME: 10 MINUTES • COOK TIME: 15 MINUTES

Veggie burgers have evolved into a classic vegetarian meal for good reason. You can avoid the higher-sodium store-bought varieties and make these simple burgers at home. Made from canned white beans and leftover rice, these burgers are quick to throw together on a weeknight, and are always handy if made in advance. Cooked veggie burgers can be frozen and reheated in the oven or toaster oven.

1 cup canned white beans, drained and rinsed

1 cup cooked white rice

1 teaspoon garlic powder

2 teaspoons dried thyme

½ teaspoon ground chipotle pepper

½ sweet onion, finely chopped

½ cup fresh or frozen corn

½ cup red bell pepper, finely chopped

Juice of 1 lemon

⅓ cup all-purpose flour

1 large egg

Freshly ground black pepper

2 teaspoons extra-virgin olive oil

1 In a large bowl, mash the beans with a potato masher, leaving a few whole beans as desired. Add the rice, garlic powder, thyme, chipotle pepper, onion, corn, bell pepper, lemon, flour, and egg, and mix well to blend. Season with pepper.

2 Using your hands, form the mixture into four patties.

3 In a large skillet over medium heat, heat the olive oil. Cook the burgers for 5 minutes, until browned on one side, flip, and cook the other side for an additional 5 minutes.

Substitution tip: Any type of canned bean can be used here, depending on your preference. Be sure to drain and rinse away the liquid, where much of the sodium lurks.

Per Serving Calories: 305; Total Fat: 4g; Saturated Fat: 1g; Cholesterol: 52mg; Carbohydrates: 57g; Fiber: 6g; Protein: 11g; Phosphorus: 181mg; Potassium: 515mg; Sodium: 281mg

Spinach Falafel Wrap

SERVES 4 • PREP TIME: 10 MINUTES • COOK TIME: 15 MINUTES

Falafel is a fun, street-food kind of sandwich filler. This spinach-loaded version, served on a tortilla, makes for an easy grab-and-go lunch that can be made up to three days in advance. The recipe makes 4 wraps, but yields about 12 extra falafels. Store these extras in an airtight container in the refrigerator or freezer, and pull them out for quick sandwiches or salad toppers.

6 ounces baby spinach

1 (15-ounce) can chickpeas, drained and rinsed

2 teaspoons ground cumin

¾ cup flour

2 tablespoons canola oil, divided, for frying

¼ cup plain, unsweetened yogurt

2 garlic cloves, minced

Juice of 1 lemon

Freshly ground black pepper

4 tortillas

1 cucumber, cut into spears

2 slices red onion

Salad greens, for serving

1. Place the spinach in a colander in the sink, and pour boiling water over it to wilt the spinach. Allow it to cool, then press as much water out of the spinach as possible.

2. In a food processor, add the spinach, chickpeas, cumin, and flour. Pulse until just blended.

3. Divide the mixture into tablespoon-size balls, and use your hands to press them flat into patties.

4. In a large skillet over medium-high heat, heat 1 tablespoon of oil. Add half of the falafel patties, and cook for 2 to 3 minutes on each side, until browned and crisp. Repeat with the remaining falafel patties.

5. In a small bowl, combine the yogurt, garlic, lemon juice, and pepper.

6. On each tortilla, place 3 falafel patties, a couple cucumber spears, a few red-onion rings, and a handful of salad greens. Top each with 1 tablespoon of the yogurt sauce.

Substitution tip: *Use other sandwich wraps, such as flatbreads or pita, if desired.*

Per Serving Calories: 241; Total Fat: 7g; Saturated Fat: 1g; Cholesterol: 2mg; Carbohydrates: 37g; Fiber: 4g; Protein: 8g; Phosphorus: 110mg; Potassium: 245mg; Sodium: 285mg

Spicy Tofu and Broccoli Stir-Fry

SERVES 4 • PREP TIME: 15 MINUTES • COOK TIME: 15 MINUTES

Tofu is easy to prepare, but squeezing out the moisture makes all the difference. When pan-frying, it is really important to expel all the moisture possible to prevent the tofu from spattering and sticking to the pan. Make squeezing the moisture out of the tofu your first step, using paper towels or a clean kitchen towel, before you prep the ingredients, and then squeeze it again right before cooking.

FOR THE SAUCE

3 garlic cloves

2-inch piece ginger, peeled

2 tablespoons honey

¼ cup rice wine vinegar

2 tablespoons
   extra-virgin olive oil

FOR THE STIR-FRY

1 (14-ounce) package
   extra-firm tofu

1 cup long-grain white rice

2 tablespoons
   extra-virgin olive oil

2 cups chopped broccoli

1 cup shredded carrots

3 scallions, finely chopped

TO MAKE THE SAUCE

Combine the garlic, ginger, honey, vinegar, and olive oil in a food processor, and purée until smooth.

TO MAKE THE STIR-FRY

1 Cut the tofu into small cubes, and press the excess moisture from the tofu using paper towels, repeating several times until dry.

2 In a medium pot, cook the rice according to package directions.

3 In a large skillet over medium heat, heat the olive oil. Add the tofu to the pan in a single layer. Carefully add one quarter of the sauce to the pan and continue to cook, flipping the tofu only once or twice every 4 minutes, until it is well browned. With a slotted spoon, transfer the tofu to a plate lined with paper towels to drain.

Continued >

Spicy Tofu and Broccoli Stir-Fry *continued*

4 Add the broccoli to the pan. Cook, covered, stirring often, until fork-tender, about 5 minutes. Add the carrots and continue to cook for an additional 3 minutes, until softened. Add the remaining sauce to the vegetables, return the tofu to the pan, and stir to mix. Garnish with scallions and serve over rice.

Substitution tip: Use an equal amount of snow peas in place of the broccoli to lower the potassium to 343mg.

Ingredient tip: You can brown your tofu in a wok, which has higher sides, to keep the oil from spattering.

Per Serving Calories: 410; Total Fat: 18g; Saturated Fat: 3g; Cholesterol: 0mg; Carbohydrates: 51g; Fiber: 4g; Protein: 13g; Phosphorus: 222mg; Potassium: 487mg; Sodium: 51mg

Tofu and Rice Salad Bowl

SERVES 4 • PREP TIME: 15 MINUTES • COOK TIME: 15 MINUTES

Baking tofu can lightly crisp its exterior without the added fat of frying. For this rice-based salad, prepare the ingredients while the tofu is baking, and you'll have a filling meal on the table in 30 minutes. Sunflower seeds contrast the soft tofu with their crunch and texture, and a mixture of shredded raw beets and carrots offers a boost of beta-carotene, magnesium, and vitamin C.

FOR THE DRESSING

2 tablespoons apple
    cider vinegar
2 garlic cloves, minced
2 tablespoons
    extra-virgin olive oil
1 tablespoon tahini
¼ cup water

FOR THE SALAD

1 (14-ounce) package
    extra-firm tofu
1 tablespoon sesame oil
1 cup white rice
4 cups mixed salad greens
1 beet, peeled and grated
2 carrots, grated
¼ cup sunflower seeds

TO MAKE THE DRESSING

In a small bowl, whisk the vinegar, garlic, olive oil, tahini, and water. Set aside.

TO MAKE THE SALAD

1 Preheat the oven to 350°F. Line a baking sheet with parchment paper.

2 Cut the tofu into bite-size rectangles about ½ inch thick. Toss with the sesame oil, and arrange in a single layer on the prepared baking sheet. Bake for 15 minutes.

3 Prepare the rice according to package directions.

4 Place a scoop of rice in each of four bowls, then top each with 1 cup of salad greens and equal portions of the beet, carrots, and sunflower seeds. Top with the baked tofu and serve with the dressing.

Cooking tip: Cook the rice in advance and store in an airtight container in the refrigerator for up to three or four days to have on hand for making quick lunches.

Per Serving Calories: 393; Total Fat: 18g; Saturated Fat: 3g; Cholesterol: 0mg; Carbohydrates: 49g; Fiber: 5g; Protein: 12g; Phosphorus: 211mg; Potassium: 362mg; Sodium: 54mg

Vegetable Biriyani

SERVES 4 • PREP TIME: 10 MINUTES • COOK TIME: 30 MINUTES

Biriyani is a South Asian rice dish featuring a mix of spices, rice, and vegetables or meat. This nutritious vegetarian version works well as either a main or side dish. If you have the time, make it the night before to allow the ingredients to meld for even more flavor.

1 cup basmati rice

2 tablespoons olive oil or butter, divided

½ teaspoon curry powder

½ teaspoon cumin seeds

½ teaspoon coriander seeds

1¾ cups water plus ⅔ cup water, divided

½ sweet onion, chopped

2 garlic cloves, minced

1 teaspoon ground coriander

½ teaspoon ground cardamom

½ teaspoon ground cumin

¼ teaspoon ground turmeric

2 cups cauliflower florets

1 cup green beans, cut into 2-inch segments

1 carrot, diced

¼ cup chopped cilantro leaves, for garnish

1. In a small bowl, rinse the rice until the water runs clear. Drain and set aside.

2. In a medium stockpot over medium heat, heat 1 tablespoon of olive oil. Add the curry powder, cumin seeds, and coriander seeds, stirring constantly, until fragrant, about 30 seconds. Add the rice to the pot along with 1¾ cups of water. Bring to a boil, reduce the heat, cover, and simmer for 12 minutes. Turn off the heat and let steam, covered, for 10 minutes.

3. In a large skillet over medium heat, heat the remaining tablespoon of olive oil. Add the onion, and cook for 6 to 8 minutes, until tender. Add the garlic and cook for an additional minute. Add the coriander, cardamom, cumin, and turmeric to the skillet, and stirring constantly, toast until fragrant, about 1 minute. Add the cauliflower, beans, and carrots, stirring to coat, and cook for 2 to 3 minutes. Add the remaining ⅔ cup of water to the pan, cover, and cook for 7 to 10 minutes, until the vegetables are just fork-tender.

4. Add the rice to the vegetables, and stir to blend. Serve topped with cilantro leaves.

Substitution tip: *Try adding 8 ounces of diced chicken in Step 3 with the onion, and proceed as directed.*

Per Serving Calories: 172; Total Fat: 4g; Saturated Fat: 1g; Cholesterol: 4mg; Carbohydrates: 31g; Fiber: 3g; Protein: 4g; Phosphorus: 40mg; Potassium: 232mg; Sodium: 23mg

Collard and Rice Stuffed Red Peppers

SERVES 4 • PREP TIME: 10 MINUTES • COOK TIME: 50 MINUTES

Stuffed peppers are the quintessential make-ahead meal—they can be prepped in advance, stored on a baking sheet covered in plastic wrap, and then heated within a day or two. Here, filling rice and health-supportive collard greens join forces for a satisfying, high-fiber meal without the meat.

2 medium red bell peppers

2 tablespoons extra-virgin olive oil, divided

Freshly ground black pepper

6 cups loosely packed collard greens, trimmed

½ sweet onion, chopped

3 garlic cloves, minced

1 cup cooked white rice

Juice of 1 lemon

¼ cup toasted sunflower seeds, divided

1   Preheat the oven to 400°F.

2   Halve the peppers through the stems, and remove the seeds and stems. Brush the inside and outside of the peppers with 1 tablespoon of olive oil and season with the pepper. Place the peppers cut-side down in a baking dish. Bake for 10 to 15 minutes, until just tender. Remove from the oven and flip the peppers cut-side up. Set aside, leaving the oven on.

3   In a large saucepan, bring 4 cups of water to a boil. Add the collard greens and cook until just tender, 5 to 7 minutes. Drain and rinse under cold water. Chop finely.

4   In a large skillet, heat the remaining tablespoon of olive oil over medium heat. Add the onion, and cook, stirring often, for 5 to 7 minutes, until it begins to brown. Add the garlic and cook until fragrant. Stir in the collard greens. Remove from the heat, and stir in the rice and lemon juice. Season with pepper.

Continued >

5 Divide the filling between the pepper halves and top each pepper half with 1 tablespoon of the sunflower seeds. Add ¼ cup of water to the baking dish, cover with aluminum foil, and bake for 20 minutes, until heated through. Uncover and bake for an additional 5 minutes.

Substitution tip: *For a milder flavor, use an equal amount of fresh spinach in place of collards.*

Per Serving Calories: 304; Total Fat: 9g; Saturated Fat: 1g; Cholesterol: 0mg; Carbohydrates: 50g; Fiber: 5g; Protein: 8g; Phosphorus: 147mg; Potassium: 397mg; Sodium: 20mg

Stuffed Delicata Squash Boats with Bulgur and Vegetables

SERVES 4 • PREP TIME: 10 MINUTES • COOK TIME: 35 MINUTES

This Tex-Mex-style stuffed squash calls upon bulgur, black beans, and corn kernels to fill the empty space in the squash and your belly. The chili powder–flavored mixture somehow makes this dish meaty tasting without any meat. And since the dish is encased in an edible squash bowl, you can eat everything, including the skin. The only caveat: Squash is quite high in potassium, so keep portion size in check—a half of a small squash is about right.

2 small delicata squash, halved lengthwise and seeded

6 teaspoons extra-virgin olive oil, divided

1 cup bulgur

½ sweet onion, diced

2 tablespoons chili powder

1 cup canned black beans, drained and rinsed

½ cup frozen or fresh corn kernels

2 scallions, thinly sliced, for garnish

1 Preheat the oven to 425°F.

2 Brush the cut squash with 2 teaspoons of olive oil and place cut-side down on a baking sheet. Cook for 25 to 30 minutes, until the flesh is tender.

3 Meanwhile, in a saucepan, bring the bulgur and 2 cups of water to a boil. Reduce the heat, cover, and simmer for 12 to 15 minutes, until the liquid is absorbed. Drain well.

4 In a large skillet, heat the remaining 4 teaspoons of olive oil over medium heat. Cook the onion for 4 to 5 minutes, until it just starts to brown. Stir in the chili powder, black beans, and corn. Stir in the bulgur, and cook for an additional minute.

5 Divide the filling between the squash halves, sprinkle with scallions, and serve.

Substitution tip: Other types of squash good for baking include butternut, buttercup, and acorn squashes—but their skins are inedible.

Per Serving Calories: 314; Total Fat: 8g; Saturated Fat: 1g; Cholesterol: 0mg; Carbohydrates: 56g; Fiber: 15g; Protein: 10g; Phosphorus: 236mg; Potassium: 812mg; Sodium: 311mg

Barley and Roasted Vegetable Bowl

SERVES 4 • PREP TIME: 10 MINUTES • COOK TIME: 30 MINUTES

The vegetable trio of eggplant, zucchini, and bell pepper is everything you could want on a summer day. Dressed with a simple lemon vinaigrette, and topped with basil and feta, this fiber-rich lunch makes for a quick anytime meal.

2 small Asian
    eggplants, diced
2 small zucchini, diced
½ red bell pepper, chopped
½ sweet onion, cut
    into wedges
2 tablespoons extra-virgin
    olive oil, divided
Freshly ground
    black pepper
1 cup barley
Juice of 1 lemon
3 garlic cloves, minced
¼ cup basil leaves,
    roughly chopped
¼ cup crumbled
    feta cheese
2 cups arugula or mixed
    baby salad greens

1 Preheat the oven to 425°F.

2 In a medium bowl, toss the eggplant, zucchini, bell pepper, and onion with 1 tablespoon of olive oil, and arrange the vegetables in a single layer on a baking sheet. Season with pepper.

3 Roast the vegetables for about 25 minutes, stirring once or twice, until they are browned and tender. Set aside.

4 Meanwhile, in a medium pot, add the barley and 2 cups of water. Bring to a boil, reduce the heat to simmer, cover, and cook for 20 minutes. Turn off the heat, and let rest for 10 minutes. Fluff with a fork, and drain any remaining water.

5 In a small bowl, whisk the lemon juice, garlic, and remaining tablespoon of olive oil.

6 Toss the vegetables with the barley, and then mix together with the lemon-garlic dressing. Right before serving, stir in the basil, feta cheese, and salad greens.

Ingredient tip: Eggplant is high in water (90 percent) and low in minerals, with one exception: potassium. Omit one eggplant to reduce the total potassium to 463mg, or omit both to reduce it to 385mg.

Per Serving Calories: 292; Total Fat: 10g; Saturated Fat: 3g; Cholesterol: 8mg; Carbohydrates: 44g; Fiber: 11g; Protein: 9g; Phosphorus: 201mg; Potassium: 543mg; Sodium: 119mg

Creamy Pesto Pasta

SERVES 4 • PREP TIME: 10 MINUTES • COOK TIME: 10 MINUTES

Basil and arugula make a spectacularly tasty pesto with a hint of herbal spiciness. Walnuts, in place of the more traditional pine nuts, provide a healthy dose of omega-3s and help support the kidneys. Linguine noodles are ideal with their ample surface area, which takes on a festive green hue when coated with this quick pesto sauce.

8 ounces linguine noodles

2 cups packed basil leaves

2 cups packed
  arugula leaves

⅓ cup walnut pieces

3 garlic cloves

¼ cup extra-virgin olive oil

Freshly ground
  black pepper

1 Fill a medium stockpot halfway with water, and bring to a boil. Cook the noodles al dente, and drain.

2 In a food processor, add the basil, arugula, walnuts, and garlic. Process until coarsely ground. With the food processor running, slowly add the olive oil, and continue to mix until creamy. Season with pepper.

3 Toss the noodles with the pesto and serve.

Substitution tip: You can swap in any type of pasta you have on hand for the linguine, and the same goes for the walnuts. Try using cashews, pistachios, pine nuts, or even sunflower seeds for a unique pesto all your own.

Per Serving Calories: 394; Total Fat: 21g; Saturated Fat: 3g; Cholesterol: 0mg; Carbohydrates: 0g; Fiber: 3g; Protein: 10g; Phosphorus: 54mg; Potassium: 148mg; Sodium: 4mg

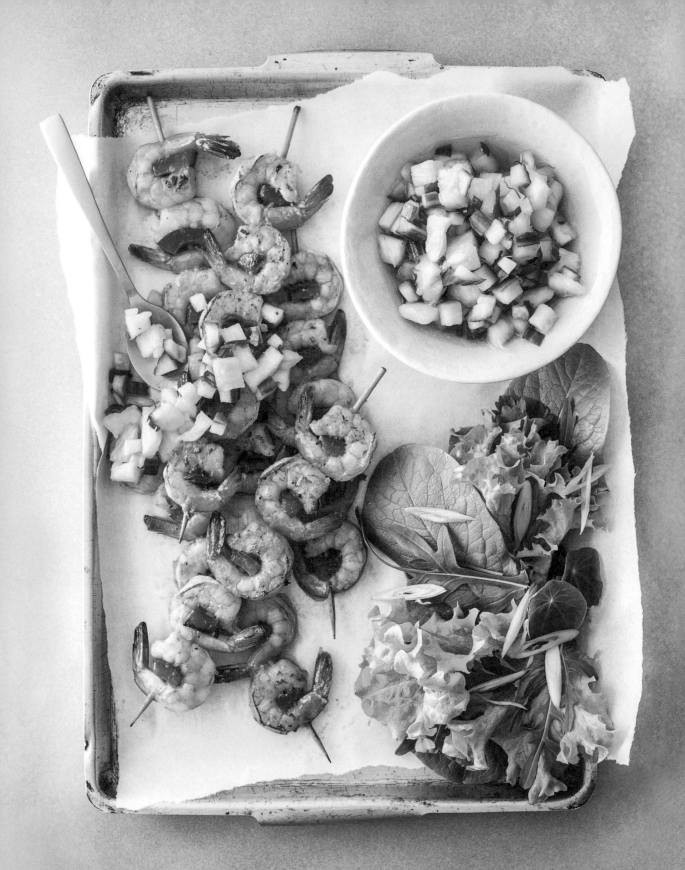

CHAPTER ELEVEN

Seafood Mains

◀ *Shrimp Skewers with Mango Cucumber Salsa, page 132*

Shrimp Skewers with Mango Cucumber Salsa

SERVES 6 • PREP TIME: 10 MINUTES, PLUS 30 MINUTES TO MARINATE
COOK TIME: 15 MINUTES

This ginger-honey-lime marinated shrimp tastes great cooked on the grill or on the stove top in a grill pan. An accompanying mango and cucumber salsa is cool and refreshing with a little bit of kick. This is one easy, festive dish that you'll want to make for dinner guests.

FOR THE SHRIMP

Juice of 2 limes

2 tablespoons honey

1-inch piece ginger, minced

1 pound large shrimp, peeled and deveined, tails intact

1 teaspoon canola oil

FOR THE SALSA

¼ cup diced sweet onion

1 small red chile, finely diced

1 medium cucumber, seeded and diced

1 mango, peeled and diced

Juice of 1 lime

TO MAKE THE SHRIMP

1 In a medium bowl, combine the lime juice, honey, and ginger. Add the shrimp and toss to coat.

2 Cover and refrigerate for 30 minutes to marinate.

3 Thread the shrimp onto skewers.

4 Heat a grill or grill pan over medium-high heat and brush with oil. Cook the skewers 3 to 6 minutes on each side, until the shrimp are opaque and cooked through.

TO MAKE THE SALSA

1 In a small bowl, toss the onion, chile, cucumber, mango, and lime juice.

2 Add the shrimp and toss to coat.

Cooking tip: If you don't have a grill pan, you can cook the skewers for 10 to 12 minutes on a rimmed baking dish in a preheated 425°F oven.

Per Serving Calories: 123; Total Fat: 2g; Saturated Fat: 0g; Cholesterol: 95mg; Carbohydrates: 17g; Fiber: 3g; Protein: 11g; Phosphorus: 213mg; Potassium: 317mg; Sodium: 431mg

Shrimp and Bok Choy in Parchment

SERVES 4 • PREP TIME: 10 MINUTES • COOK TIME: 15 MINUTES

Seafood cooked in parchment paper is the answer to a busy night. The simple packets can be prepared the day before, leaving you to just turn on the oven and pop them in when you get home. Ginger and sesame oil elevate this lively meal, and a generous portion of bok choy makes it as filling as it is delicious.

12 ounces shrimp, peeled and deveined

3 garlic cloves, minced

2-inch piece ginger, minced

1 teaspoon toasted sesame oil

2 teaspoons honey

2 tablespoons freshly squeezed lime juice

2 tablespoons rice vinegar

1 pound bok choy, white and green parts thinly sliced

2 scallions, thinly sliced

1 jalapeño pepper, thinly sliced

¼ cup chopped cilantro

1 Preheat the oven to 375°F.

2 In a small bowl, mix the shrimp, garlic, and ginger.

3 In another small bowl, stir together the sesame oil, honey, lime juice, and rice vinegar.

4 Cut four large circles, 12 inches in diameter, of parchment paper. On each piece, place a large handful of bok choy, and top with the shrimp and garlic-ginger mixture, scallions, and jalapeño slices. Drizzle each pile with one quarter of the vinegar–lime juice mixture.

5 Fold the parchment paper in half, creating a half-moon shape. Fold the edges together to create a seal.

6 Place the packets on a rimmed baking sheet and cook for 15 minutes. Remove from the oven and let rest for 5 minutes before serving. When opening the packet, watch for escaping steam. Garnish with cilantro and serve with white rice.

Substitution tip: *Bok choy is ideal because it is quick to cook, and the stems and leaves add texture. However, green cabbage or Napa cabbage can be used in its place.*

Per Serving Calories: 92; Total Fat: 2g; Saturated Fat: 0g; Cholesterol: 107mg; Carbohydrates: 6g; Fiber: 1g; Protein: 12g; Phosphorus: 217mg; Potassium: 162mg; Sodium: 484mg

Shrimp Fried Rice

SERVES 6 • PREP TIME: 10 MINUTES • COOK TIME: 15 MINUTES

Restaurant-style fried rice is loaded with soy sauce, which is very high in sodium and can wreak havoc on your body. This simple fried rice uses garlic, ginger, and onion to pack in authentic flavor. Make it on a weeknight using cold leftover rice, which handles best when making fried rice, and you'll have dinner on the table in under 30 minutes.

1 tablespoon
  extra-virgin olive oil
½ sweet onion, chopped
2-inch piece ginger, minced
3 garlic cloves, minced
1 pound shrimp, peeled
  and deveined
1 cup sugar snap peas
3 cups cooked rice

1 In a large skillet or wok over medium heat, heat the oil.

2 Add the onion and cook, stirring continuously, for 3 to 5 minutes, until it softens.

3 Add the ginger and garlic, and stir until just fragrant.

4 Add the shrimp and cook, stirring often, for about 5 minutes, until the shrimp is opaque and nearly cooked through.

5 Stir in the snap peas and rice, stirring until mixed well and heated through. Serve.

Substitution tip: *Add your favorite vegetables or explore some new ones to make this dish your own. Broccoli stems, jicama, or daikon cut into matchsticks add a nice flavor, as do carrots, eggplant, and peas. For even more flavor, add a handful of chopped cilantro or basil to the pan at the end of cooking.*

Per Serving Calories: 217; Total Fat: 3g; Saturated Fat: 1g; Cholesterol: 95mg; Carbohydrates: 32g; Fiber: 1g; Protein: 13g; Phosphorus: 226mg; Potassium: 157mg; Sodium: 431mg

Creamy Shrimp Fettuccine

SERVES 4 • PREP TIME: 10 MINUTES • COOK TIME: 30 MINUTES

Creamy pasta can still be enjoyed, even on a renal diet. It simply requires a few creative substitutions for some of its higher-fat ingredients, and you'll create a comforting and satisfying bowl of shrimp fettuccine in pretty short order!

8 ounces dried fettuccine

2 tablespoons extra-virgin olive oil, divided

10 ounces shrimp, peeled and deveined

3 garlic cloves, minced

2 tablespoons all-purpose flour

1 cup Homemade Rice Milk (page 70) or unsweetened store-bought rice milk

1 teaspoon garlic powder

¼ cup grated Parmesan cheese

Freshly ground black pepper

2 tablespoons chopped parsley

Lemon, cut into wedges, for serving

1. Bring a large stockpot of salted water to a boil. Add the fettuccine, and cook the noodles, stirring occasionally, until al dente. Drain.

2. In a large skillet over medium heat, heat 1 tablespoon of olive oil. Add the shrimp and cook, stirring occasionally, for 3 to 5 minutes, until they turn pink and opaque. Using a slotted spoon, remove the shrimp from the pan, and set aside.

3. Add the remaining tablespoon of oil to the skillet. Add the garlic, and cook until fragrant. Add the flour, and mix until it comes together as a paste.

4. Add the rice milk slowly, a little at a time, whisking continuously, until it is all added and the mixture is smooth. Stir in the garlic powder. Reduce the heat and let simmer for 3 to 4 minutes, until the sauce begins to thicken. Stir in the Parmesan cheese. Season with pepper.

5. Add the noodles and stir to coat. Stir in the shrimp. Serve garnished with parsley and lemon wedges.

Substitution tip: This is an infinitely customizable dish. Swap out the shrimp for chicken, or make it vegetarian instead by adding fresh green peas or snow peas to the skillet with the garlic powder in Step 4.

Per Serving Calories: 379; Total Fat: 11g; Saturated Fat: 2g; Cholesterol: 95mg; Carbohydrates: 52g; Fiber: 3g; Protein: 20g; Phosphorus: 233mg; Potassium: 141mg; Sodium: 527mg

Lemon Garlic Halibut

SERVES 4 • PREP TIME: 10 MINUTES, PLUS UP TO 1 HOUR TO MARINATE
COOK TIME: 15 MINUTES

Sometimes the simplest flavorings are just enough to really set off a piece of fish. These humble halibut fillets stand out when baked in this lemon-and-garlic marinade, and topped with fresh herbs. For the most tender and noteworthy results, cook the fish until it just flakes.

¼ cup freshly squeezed
lemon juice

2 tablespoons extra-virgin
olive oil, divided

2 garlic cloves, minced

Freshly ground
black pepper

1 pound halibut fillets,
skin removed

Zest of 1 lemon

2 tablespoons chopped
fresh cilantro

2 tablespoons chopped
fresh parsley

1   Preheat the oven to 400°F.

2   In a medium bowl, mix the lemon juice, 1 tablespoon of olive oil, and garlic. Season with pepper. Add the halibut fillets, flipping them once or twice to coat. Refrigerate for 10 minutes to marinate.

3   Arrange the fillets on a baking sheet and brush with the marinade. Cook for 12 to 15 minutes, brushing with the marinade once about halfway through. Cook until the fish flakes with a fork. Discard the marinade, and serve the fish topped with lemon zest, cilantro, and parsley.

Cooking tip: *Just 10 minutes in, the marinade will infuse the fish with plenty of flavor, but you can marinate the fish for up to 1 hour beforehand.*

Per Serving Calories: 169; Total Fat: 8g; Saturated Fat: 1g; Cholesterol: 56mg; Carbohydrates: 2g; Fiber: 0g; Protein: 21g; Phosphorus: 272mg; Potassium: 528mg; Sodium: 79mg

White Fish and Broccoli Curry

SERVES 6 • PREP TIME: 10 MINUTES • COOK TIME: 10 MINUTES

A traditional Thai curry uses coconut milk, but because coconut milk is so high in phosphorus, this recipe substitutes a blend of rice milk and cream cheese to create a similarly rich and smooth curry. Blend the curry paste up to a day in advance, and this quick curry will be ready to go the moment hunger strikes.

FOR THE CURRY PASTE

½ sweet onion, chopped

1 medium red
   chile, chopped

1-inch piece ginger,
   peeled and chopped

1 lemongrass stalk, outer
   leaves removed, tender
   bottom portion chopped

¼ cup roughly chopped
   fresh cilantro stems

1 teaspoon
   turmeric powder

½ teaspoon cumin seeds

2 tablespoons
   extra-virgin olive oil

FOR THE CURRY

¾ cup Homemade
   Rice Milk (page 70)
   or unsweetened
   store-bought rice milk

½ cup cream cheese

1 pound tilapia fillets

3 cups broccoli florets

Juice of 1 lime

1 teaspoon sugar

TO MAKE THE CURRY PASTE

Using a mortar and pestle or blender, combine the onion, chile, ginger, lemongrass, cilantro, turmeric, cumin seeds, and olive oil, and blend until smooth.

TO MAKE THE CURRY

1 In a large skillet over medium-high heat, heat the curry paste, and cook, stirring occasionally, for 2 to 3 minutes, until fragrant. Add the rice milk and stir until incorporated. Bring to a light simmer.

2 Meanwhile, in a small bowl, add the cream cheese. Add a few tablespoons of the hot rice-milk mixture and stir until blended.

3 Add the tilapia and broccoli to the skillet, then add the cream-cheese mixture, gently stirring to blend.

4 Cook for 3 to 5 minutes, until the fish is cooked through, the broccoli is fork-tender, and the curry is bubbly. Stir in the lime juice and sugar. Remove from the heat, and serve over white rice.

Substitution tip: *Instead of tilapia, you can use other similar white fish, such as catfish or flounder. Be sure to remove any pin bones in fillets before cooking.*

Per Serving Calories: 223; Total Fat: 13g; Saturated Fat: 5g; Cholesterol: 59mg; Carbohydrates: 10g; Fiber: 2g; Protein: 18g; Phosphorus: 194mg; Potassium: 490mg; Sodium: 134mg

Oven-Fried Fish
with Pineapple Salsa

SERVES 4 • PREP TIME: 10 MINUTES • COOK TIME: 20 MINUTES

Who doesn't love fried fish? Only that the high fat content can make it prohibitive for a healthy diet, but here's good news—you can still achieve that great crisp crust without frying. This dish employs a smart technique to bake the crispiness into the fish. Seasoned generously with garlic powder, this browned breaded fish gets crowned with a sweet and spicy salsa topping.

FOR THE PINEAPPLE SALSA

1 cup diced pineapple

¼ cup diced red onion

½ jalapeño pepper,
   seeded and diced

Juice of ½ lime

¼ cup chopped
   fresh cilantro

FOR THE FISH

1 tablespoon butter

1 pound white fish fillets,
   such as tilapia or whiting

½ teaspoon garlic powder

½ teaspoon paprika

¼ cup yellow cornmeal

¼ cup all-purpose flour

1 egg, beaten

2 tablespoons Homemade
   Rice Milk (page 70)
   or unsweetened
   store-bought rice milk

FOR THE SALSA

In a small bowl, combine the pineapple, onion, jalapeño, lime juice, and cilantro. Toss and set aside while you make the fish.

FOR THE FISH

1 Preheat the oven to 400°F. Butter a small baking dish.

2 Season the fish fillets with garlic powder and paprika.

3 In a small bowl, mix the cornmeal and flour.

4 In another small bowl, mix the egg and rice milk.

5 Dip each piece of fish in the egg mixture, and next roll in the flour mixture. Place the fish in a single layer in the prepared pan. Bake for 20 minutes, flipping once halfway through, until the fish is golden and flakes easily with a fork.

Cooking tip: For the crispiest crust, be sure to wait until a nice golden crust has formed on the underside of the fish in the baking dish before flipping.

Per Serving Calories: 242; Total Fat: 7g; Saturated Fat: 3g; Cholesterol: 116mg; Carbohydrates: 20g; Fiber: 1g; Protein: 27g; Phosphorus: 238mg; Potassium: 474mg; Sodium: 83mg

Salmon and Kale in Parchment

SERVES 4 • PREP TIME: 10 MINUTES • COOK TIME: 15 MINUTES

This no-fuss meal comes together in minutes, and once you get it in the oven, you can sit back and relax until dinner is done. Seasoned with thyme, rosemary, and lemon, this salmon dish is fragrant and tender, and when served with white rice, everything balances out to a tasty and satisfying meal.

2 cups thinly sliced
   kale leaves

2 small zucchini, sliced

Freshly ground
   black pepper

1 pound salmon fillets

½ teaspoon paprika

4 fresh rosemary sprigs

4 fresh thyme sprigs

1 lemon, sliced

¼ cup dry white wine

1   Preheat the oven to 450°F.

2   Cut four pieces of parchment paper, each about 12 inches in diameter.

3   On each paper, lay ½ cup of kale leaves, topped with several slices of zucchini. Season with pepper.

4   Season the salmon fillets with paprika, then top each fillet with a thyme sprig, a rosemary sprig, and a slice of lemon. Pour 1 tablespoon of white wine over each fillet.

5   Fold the parchment paper over to join the seams, and crease to form a seal.

6   Bake for 15 minutes. Remove from the oven and let the fillets cool for about 5 minutes before serving.

Substitution tip: In place of the kale, use collard green leaves, with the tough stems removed, to cut the potassium in the dish to 494mg.

Per Serving Calories: 201; Total Fat: 7g; Saturated Fat: 1g; Cholesterol: 60mg; Carbohydrates: 60g; Fiber: 2g; Protein: 26g; Phosphorus: 332mg; Potassium: 614mg; Sodium: 144mg

Salmon Burgers

SERVES 4 • PREP TIME: 10 MINUTES • COOK TIME: 10 MINUTES

Opt for fresh salmon in this fun dish, so you don't have to worry about the extra sodium inside canned salmon. Raw salmon is great because it gets pasty and easily holds together without additional binders. Lemon juice and zest brighten the fish, and bread crumbs help it crisp nicely for a superb salmon burger from scratch.

1 pound boneless, skinless salmon

1 tablespoon Dijon mustard

Zest of 1 lemon

1 tablespoon freshly squeezed lemon juice

Freshly ground black pepper

2 scallions, sliced

½ cup coarse bread crumbs, divided

1 tablespoon extra-virgin olive oil

Buns or greens, for serving

1 Remove any pin bones, and cut the salmon into chunks. In a food processor, add half the salmon, and pulse until pasty. Add the mustard, lemon zest, and lemon juice. Season with pepper.

2 Transfer the fish mixture to a bowl. Stir in the scallions and ¼ cup of bread crumbs. Form into four patties. Spread the remaining bread crumbs on a plate, and press each patty into the bread crumbs to lightly coat.

3 In a large skillet over medium-high heat, heat the olive oil. Add the burgers and cook for 3 to 4 minutes, then flip and cook the other side for 2 to 3 minutes. Serve on a bun or over a bed of greens, such as Mixed Green Leaf and Citrus Salad (page 109) or Spinach Salad with Orange Vinaigrette (page 108).

Cooking tip: *Make the burgers up to a few hours ahead, and refrigerate them in an airtight container until ready for use.*

Per Serving Calories: 224; Total Fat: 5g; Saturated Fat: 1g; Cholesterol: 52mg; Carbohydrates: 19g; Fiber: 1g; Protein: 25g; Phosphorus: 304mg; Potassium: 499mg; Sodium: 209mg

Roasted Salmon with Herb Gremolata

SERVES 4 • PREP TIME: 10 MINUTES • COOK TIME: 15 MINUTES

The great thing about using plenty of herbs in your cooking is that they effectively make up for the absence of table salt, providing an incredible and surprising depth. The herbal gremolata smothered over this fish before cooking combines thyme, rosemary, garlic, and lemon juice, providing robust flavor to the mild, flaky salmon. Serve with white rice.

½ cup loosely packed, finely chopped parsley leaves

Zest and juice of 1 lemon

2 garlic cloves, minced

1 tablespoon chopped fresh rosemary

1 tablespoon chopped fresh thyme

1 pound skinless salmon fillets

Freshly ground black pepper

1 Preheat the oven to 400°F.

2 In a small bowl, add the parsley, lemon zest, lemon juice, garlic, rosemary, and thyme. Stir to blend.

3 Press the fillets into the herb mixture to coat on one side, and place them herb-side up on a baking sheet. Season with pepper. Cook for 12 minutes, until the fish is just cooked and flakes with a fork.

Substitution tip: *This same gremolata tastes great on other types of fish, including white fish as well as other fatty fish. You can also play around with the gremolata, adding other herbs that you have on hand, such as cilantro, mint, or sage.*

Per Serving Calories: 170; Total Fat: 7g; Saturated Fat: 1g; Cholesterol: 62mg; Carbohydrates: 2g; Fiber: 1g; Protein: 23g; Phosphorus: 236mg; Potassium: 626mg; Sodium: 55mg

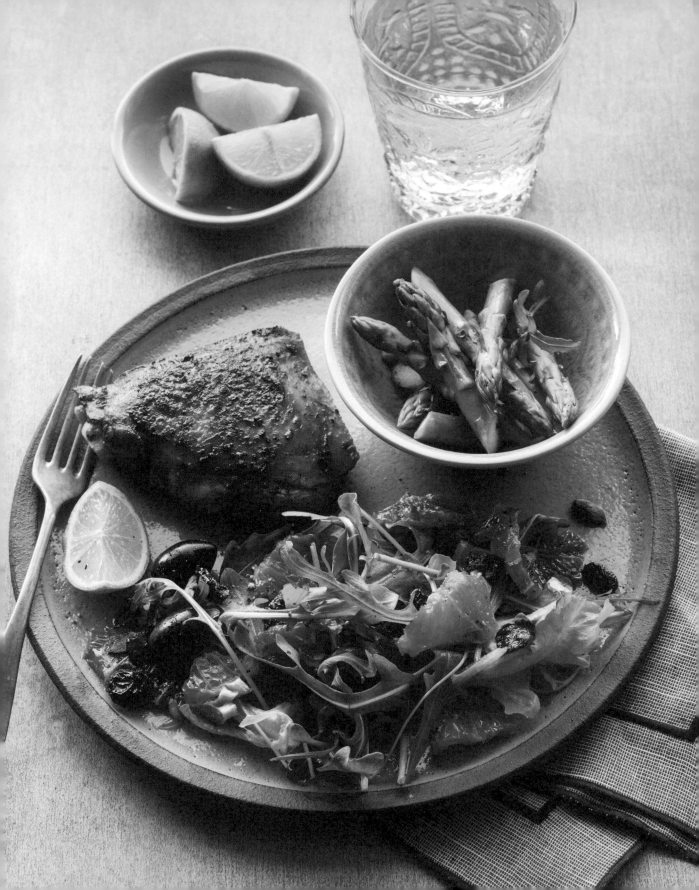

CHAPTER TWELVE

Poultry and Meat Mains

◀ *One-Pan Curried Chicken Thighs and Cauliflower, page 152*

Chicken Kebab Sandwich

SERVES 4 • PREP TIME: 15 MINUTES • COOK TIME: 15 MINUTES

If you are a fan of this street-food classic, look no further than your kitchen to enjoy this perennial favorite. Simple to make and overflowing with flavor, this sandwich comes together in just a few minutes if you prep the meat the night before. In fact, you can prep the yogurt sauce and chicken up to three days ahead.

12 ounces boneless, skinless chicken breast

2 tablespoons freshly squeezed lemon juice

1 tablespoon extra-virgin olive oil

4 garlic cloves, minced, divided

Freshly ground black pepper

¼ cup plain, unsweetened yogurt

4 white flatbreads

1 cucumber, sliced

1 cup lettuce, shredded

1 In a medium bowl, add the chicken breast, lemon juice, olive oil, and half the garlic, tossing to coat. Season with pepper. Set aside to marinate while you prepare the other ingredients.

2 In a small bowl, add the yogurt and remaining garlic. Season with pepper and mix well. Set aside.

3 Heat a large skillet over medium-high heat, and add the chicken and the marinade. Cook for 5 minutes, until the chicken is well browned on the underside. Flip it over and cook the other side until the chicken is golden brown and the juices run clear. Remove from the pan and let rest for 5 minutes. Cut the chicken into thin slices.

4 In each flatbread, add some chicken, cucumber, and lettuce. Top with the yogurt sauce, and serve.

Lower sodium tip: *Reduce the amount of chicken breast to 8 ounces to lower this dish to 275mg and 15g of protein.*

Per Serving Calories: 217; Total Fat: 6g; Saturated Fat: 1g; Cholesterol: 49mg; Carbohydrates: 21g; Fiber: 1g; Protein: 22g; Phosphorus: 80mg; Potassium: 231mg; Sodium: 339mg

Aromatic Chicken and Cabbage Stir-Fry

SERVES 4 • PREP TIME: 10 MINUTES • COOK TIME: 10 MINUTES

Cabbage tops the charts as one of the world's healthiest vegetables, boasting more vitamin C than oranges, plus lots of calcium and vitamin E. Unfortunately, it sometimes gets a bad rap for its sulfuric odor and its propensity to cause intestinal gas. Utilize a secret to success with cabbage: Cook it lightly until just tender and sweet to avoid these negative attributes.

1 teaspoon canola oil

10 ounces boneless, skinless chicken breast, thinly sliced

3 cups green cabbage, thinly sliced

1 tablespoon cornstarch

1 teaspoon ground ginger

½ teaspoon garlic powder

¼ cup water

Freshly ground black pepper

1   In a large skillet over medium-high heat, heat the oil. Add the chicken and cook, stirring often, until browned and cooked through.

2   Add the cabbage to the pan, and cook for another 2 to 3 minutes, until the cabbage is tender but still crisp and green.

3   In a small bowl, mix the cornstarch, ginger, garlic, and water. Add the mixture to the pan, and continue cooking until the sauce has slightly thickened, about 1 minute. Season with pepper.

Substitution tip: *Collards, turnip greens, or mustard greens can be used in this stir-fry in place of cabbage. Because the cooking time is short, remove any tough stems to ensure even cooking.*

Per Serving Calories: 96; Total Fat: 2g; Saturated Fat: 0g; Cholesterol: 38mg; Carbohydrates: 5g; Fiber: 1g; Protein: 15g; Phosphorus: 15mg; Potassium: 140mg; Sodium: 156mg

Chicken Chow Mein

SERVES 6 • PREP TIME: 10 MINUTES • COOK TIME: 15 MINUTES

Ah, comfort food at its finest. Chicken, cabbage, carrots, and bean sprouts come together in this simple stir-fry, which can be on the table in under 30 minutes. Sesame oil and low-sodium soy sauce create a rich and flavorful combination that, when mixed with a generous portion of noodles, helps you feel cozy and satiated on a draining day.

2 teaspoons cornstarch

1 tablespoon water

1 teaspoon low-sodium
  soy sauce

1 teaspoon rice wine

1 teaspoon sugar

1 teaspoon sesame oil

2 teaspoons canola oil

3 garlic cloves, minced

8 ounces boneless,
  skinless chicken
  thighs, thinly sliced

2 cups shredded
  green cabbage

1 carrot, julienned

4 scallions, cut into
  2-inch pieces

10 ounces chow mein
  noodles, cooked
  according to
  package directions

1 cup mung bean sprouts

1 In a small bowl, mix the cornstarch, water, and soy sauce. Stir in the rice wine, sugar, and sesame oil, mixing well. Set aside.

2 In a large skillet or wok over medium-high heat, heat the canola oil.

3 Add the garlic, and cook until just fragrant, stirring constantly. Add the chicken, and cook for 1 minute, stirring, until the chicken is browned but not cooked through.

4 Add the cabbage, carrot, and scallions, and cook for 1 to 2 minutes, until the cabbage begins to wilt and the chicken is cooked through.

5 Add the noodles, and toss with the chicken and vegetables. Pour in the sauce, and stir to coat. Add the bean sprouts, and stir. Remove from the heat, and serve.

Serving tip: Test out your chopsticks skills with this recipe. It's fun to do and will also slow down the dining ritual to the ceremony it deserves.

Per Serving Calories: 342; Total Fat: 18g; Saturated Fat: 3g; Cholesterol: 31mg; Carbohydrates: 34g; Fiber: 3g; Protein: 13g; Phosphorus: 169mg; Potassium: 308mg; Sodium: 289 mg

Baked Herbed Chicken

SERVES 6 • PREP TIME: 10 MINUTES • COOK TIME: 40 MINUTES

Baking chicken is probably one of the easiest things you can do in your kitchen. It is a nearly hands-off task that makes it easy to get winning results. This recipe calls for chicken thighs, which tend to be very inexpensive yet are juicier than breast meat and nearly as meaty. Pair this aromatic, skin-on chicken with Vegetable Couscous (page 90) or with any salad for a quick and delicious meal.

4 tablespoons butter, at room temperature

4 garlic cloves, minced

1 tablespoon chopped fresh oregano

1 tablespoon chopped fresh parsley

1 teaspoon lemon zest

6 bone-in chicken thighs

¼ teaspoon freshly ground black pepper

1 Preheat the oven to 425°F.

2 In a small bowl, add the butter, garlic, oregano, parsley, and lemon zest. Mix well.

3 Arrange the thighs on a baking tray, and gently peel back the skin, leaving it attached. Brush the thigh meat with a couple of teaspoons of the butter mixture, and replace the skin to cover the meat. Season with pepper.

4 Bake for 40 minutes, until the skin is crisp and the juices run clear. Let rest for 5 minutes before serving.

Cooking tip: To reduce the total fat per serving to just 9g, remove and discard the skin after cooking.

Per Serving Calories: 226; Total Fat: 17g; Saturated Fat: 8g; Cholesterol: 78mg; Carbohydrates: 1g; Fiber: 0g; Protein: 16g; Phosphorus: 114mg; Potassium: 158mg; Sodium: 120mg

Thai-Style Chicken Curry

SERVES 4 • PREP TIME: 15 MINUTES • COOK TIME: 15 MINUTES

Most Thai curries use coconut milk, but this curry is an exception. Made in the style of a jungle curry, it uses herbs and spices alone to create a complex curry. Spicy and delicious, this dish originated in forested areas of Thailand, where coconuts are not common. Serve this dish over rice to cut the heat.

FOR THE CURRY PASTE

2 dried Thai red chiles

2 teaspoons coriander seeds

1 lemongrass stalk, outer layer removed, ends trimmed, tender green and white parts minced

1 shallot

4 garlic cloves

2-inch piece ginger, thinly sliced

½ cup coarsely chopped fresh cilantro leaves and stems

1 teaspoon low-sodium soy sauce

2 tablespoons lime juice

TO MAKE THE CURRY PASTE

1   In a small bowl, add the chiles and cover with hot water. Leave to soak for 10 minutes.

2   Meanwhile, in a small, dry skillet, toast the coriander seeds until fragrant, shaking the pan constantly to prevent burning. Transfer immediately to a food processor.

3   Drain the chiles and add them to the food processor, then add the lemongrass, shallot, garlic, ginger, cilantro, soy sauce, and lime juice. Grind into a fine paste, adding 1 or 2 tablespoons of water if needed. Use immediately, or transfer to an airtight container and store refrigerated for up to three days.

FOR THE CURRY

1 teaspoon canola oil

1 pound boneless,
skinless chicken
breast, thinly sliced

1 cup green beans, cut
into 2-inch segments

1 cup water

Juice of 1 lime

1 teaspoon brown sugar

TO MAKE THE CURRY

1 In a large skillet or wok over medium-high heat, heat the oil. Add the curry paste, and cook, stirring constantly, for about 30 seconds, until fragrant. Add the chicken breast, and stir continuously until just browned.

2 Add the beans and 1 cup of water. Simmer for 5 minutes, until the chicken is cooked through and the vegetables are tender.

3 Season with the lime juice and brown sugar. Serve over rice or rice noodles.

Lower sodium tip: Cut the soy sauce from the curry paste to reduce sodium to 236mg.

Per Serving Calories: 149; Total Fat: 3g; Saturated Fat: 1g; Cholesterol: 60mg; Carbohydrates: 9g; Fiber: 2g; Protein: 25g; Phosphorus: 35mg; Potassium: 205mg; Sodium: 280mg

Chicken Satay with Peanut Sauce

SERVES 6 • PREP TIME: 10 MINUTES, PLUS 2 HOURS TO MARINATE
COOK TIME: 10 MINUTES

Originally from Indonesia, but today a universal street-fair favorite, satay is simply grilled and skewered meat served with sauce. This recipe minimizes the sodium while still delivering intense flavor and complexity. Serve the chicken with crisp lettuce, rice, and the accompanying peanut sauce for a complete meal.

FOR THE CHICKEN

½ cup plain, unsweetened yogurt

2 garlic cloves, minced

1-inch piece ginger, minced

2 teaspoons curry powder

1 pound boneless, skinless chicken breast, cut into strips

1 teaspoon canola oil

FOR THE PEANUT SAUCE

¾ cup smooth unsalted peanut butter

1 teaspoon soy sauce

1 tablespoon brown sugar

Juice of 2 limes

½ teaspoon red chili flakes

¼ cup hot water

Fresh cilantro leaves, chopped, for garnish

Lime wedges, for garnish

TO MAKE THE CHICKEN

1 In a small bowl, add the yogurt, garlic, ginger, and curry powder. Stir to mix. Add the chicken strips to the marinade. Cover and refrigerate for 2 hours.

2 Thread the chicken pieces onto skewers.

3 Brush a grill pan with the oil, and heat on medium-high. Cook the chicken skewers on each side for 3 to 5 minutes, until cooked through.

TO MAKE THE PEANUT SAUCE

In a food processor, combine the peanut butter, soy sauce, brown sugar, lime juice, red chili flakes, and hot water. Process until smooth. Transfer to a bowl, and sprinkle with the cilantro. Serve with the chicken satay along with lime wedges for squeezing over the skewers.

Cooking tip: Metal skewers are ideal, as they require little preparation. If you have wood skewers, soak them for at least 30 minutes before cooking to prevent burning.

Per Serving Calories: 286; Total Fat: 18g; Saturated Fat: 4g; Cholesterol: 43mg; Carbohydrates: 10g; Fiber: 3g; Protein: 25g; Phosphorus: 33mg; Potassium: 66mg; Sodium: 201mg

Chicken Breast and Bok Choy in Parchment

SERVES 4 • PREP TIME: 10 MINUTES • COOK TIME: 30 MINUTES

Just like fish in parchment, chicken in parchment stands out as a quick and impressive meal that requires little effort. These can be assembled the night before and refrigerated until you walk in the door from work. Turn on the oven, throw them in, and sit back and put your feet up until dinner is ready.

1 tablespoon
Dijon mustard

1 tablespoon
extra-virgin olive oil

1 tablespoon chopped
fresh thyme leaves

2 cups thinly sliced
bok choy

2 carrots, julienned

1 small leek, thinly sliced

4 boneless, skinless
chicken breasts

Freshly ground
black pepper

4 lemon slices

1 Preheat the oven to 425°F.

2 In a small bowl, mix the mustard, olive oil, and thyme.

3 Prepare four pieces of parchment paper by folding four 18-inch pieces in half and cutting them like you would to create a heart. Open each piece and lay flat.

4 In each piece of parchment, arrange ½ cup of bok choy, a small handful of carrots, and a few slices of leek. Place the chicken breast on top, and season with pepper.

5 Brush the marinade over the chicken breasts, and top each with a slice of lemon.

6 Fold the packets shut, and fold the paper along the edges to crease and seal the packages.

7 Cook for 20 minutes. Let rest for 5 minutes, and open carefully to serve.

Substitution tip: *Bok choy works especially well in parchment, but any greens you have on hand can be substituted, as well as other vegetables, like sugar snap peas, asparagus, or broccoli.*

Per Serving Calories: 164; Total Fat: 5g; Saturated Fat: 1g; Cholesterol: 60mg; Carbohydrates: 8g; Fiber: 2g; Protein: 24g; Phosphorus: 26mg; Potassium: 187mg; Sodium: 356mg

One-Pan Curried Chicken Thighs and Cauliflower

SERVES 6 • PREP TIME: 10 MINUTES, PLUS 2 HOURS TO MARINATE
COOK TIME: 40 MINUTES

Your kitchen will smell wonderful as this one-tray delight sizzles in the oven with its rich aroma of cumin and curry. The hearty cauliflower can stand up on its own with the chicken for a meal, or you can pair it with rice or a salad if you need a bit more to keep you going.

3 tablespoons
  curry powder
½ teaspoon ground cumin
¼ teaspoon paprika
½ teaspoon freshly ground
  black pepper, divided
6 bone-in chicken thighs
4 teaspoons extra-virgin
  olive oil, divided
1 cauliflower head,
  cut into florets
½ teaspoon dried oregano
Juice of 2 limes

1. In a small bowl, mix the curry powder, cumin, paprika, and ¼ teaspoon of pepper.

2. In a medium bowl, drizzle 2 teaspoons of olive oil over the chicken thighs, and sprinkle with the curry mixture. Cover, refrigerate, and marinate for at least 2 hours or up to overnight.

3. Preheat the oven to 400°F.

4. In a medium bowl, toss the cauliflower with the remaining 2 teaspoons of olive oil and the oregano. In a single layer, arrange the chicken and cauliflower on a baking sheet.

5. Bake for 40 minutes, stirring the cauliflower and flipping the chicken pieces once during cooking, until the chicken is well browned and its juices run clear.

6. Drizzle with the lime juice and serve.

Substitution tip: Broccoli or asparagus can be used in place of cauliflower.

Per Serving Calories: 175; Total Fat: 10g; Saturated Fat: 2g; Cholesterol: 50mg; Carbohydrates: 8g; Fiber: 3g; Protein: 16g; Phosphorus: 152mg; Potassium: 486mg; Sodium: 77mg

Asian-Style Pan-Fried Chicken

SERVES 4 • PREP TIME: 20 MINUTES • COOK TIME: 25 MINUTES

When marinated in low-sodium soy sauce, rice wine, and fresh ginger, these chicken pieces take on a deliciously subtle flavor. Cornstarch breading coats the meat with a crisp exterior, but it can easily burn, so keep a close watch as it cooks. Serve these chicken pieces with plain white rice and steamed broccoli for a simple, pleasing meal.

12 ounces boneless, skinless chicken thighs, fat removed, cut into 2 or 3 pieces each

1 teaspoon low-sodium soy sauce

1 teaspoon dry rice wine

1-inch piece ginger, minced

½ cup cornstarch

3 teaspoons canola oil, divided

1 lemon, cut into wedges

1 In a medium bowl, combine the chicken, soy sauce, rice wine, and ginger. Toss and let sit for 15 minutes.

2 Toss the chicken again, and drain the liquid from the bowl. One at a time, dip the chicken pieces in the cornstarch to coat.

3 In a medium skillet over medium-high heat, heat 1½ teaspoons of oil. Add half of the chicken to the pan, and cook until golden brown on one side, about 3 to 5 minutes. Flip, and continue to cook on the opposite side, until the chicken is cooked through and is golden brown. Transfer the chicken to a plate lined with paper towels to cool. Add the remaining 1½ teaspoons of oil, and repeat the cooking process with the remaining chicken thighs.

4 Serve garnished with lemon wedges.

Substitution tip: If you don't have cornstarch, use all-purpose flour in its place. However, you may need to cook the chicken a minute or two longer to create that nice browned and crisp coating.

Per Serving Calories: 198; Total Fat: 7g; Saturated Fat: 1g; Cholesterol: 71mg; Carbohydrates: 16g; Fiber: 0g; Protein: 17g; Phosphorus: 148mg; Potassium: 218mg; Sodium: 119mg

Chicken, Pasta, and Broccoli Bake

SERVES 6 • PREP TIME: 5 MINUTES • COOK TIME: 30 MINUTES

Casseroles pack an entire meal into themselves, and this one comes out vegetable-rich and satisfying. Gather the ingredients for this creamy chicken and broccoli bake, and dinner will be on the table in about 30 minutes. Leftovers are great reheated.

8 ounces egg noodles

1 (10-ounce) package broccoli florets

2 tablespoons butter

½ sweet onion, chopped

¼ cup all-purpose flour

1½ cups Simple Chicken Broth (page 180) or low-sodium store-bought chicken stock

Freshly ground black pepper

¾ cup Homemade Rice Milk (page 70) or unsweetened store-bought rice milk

3 cups shredded cooked chicken breast

¼ cup shredded Cheddar cheese

1 Preheat the oven to 350°F. Grease a 2-quart baking dish.

2 Fill a large pot with water and bring to a boil. Add the egg noodles and cook for 5 minutes. Add the broccoli and continue to cook for 3 to 5 more minutes, until the noodles are tender and the broccoli is just fork-tender. Drain and set aside.

3 In a medium saucepan over medium-high heat, heat the butter. Add the onion and cook for 3 to 5 minutes, until it begins to soften. Add the flour and stir until evenly mixed. Add the broth and season with pepper. Simmer for 5 minutes, until it begins to thicken. Add the rice milk and cook until heated through.

4 Toss the sauce with the broccoli, noodles, and cooked chicken, and transfer to the prepared baking dish. Top with the Cheddar cheese.

5 Bake for 20 minutes, uncovered, until browned and bubbly.

Cooking tip: To make this dish in advance, complete steps 2 through 4, cover, and refrigerate overnight. The following day, bake for 30 minutes in the greased baking dish in a preheated oven.

Per Serving Calories: 351; Total Fat: 11g; Saturated Fat: 5g; Cholesterol: 86mg; Carbohydrates: 38g; Fiber: 3g; Protein: 24g; Phosphorus: 271mg; Potassium: 402mg; Sodium: 152mg

Turkey Meatballs and Spaghetti in Garlic Sauce

SERVES 4 • PREP TIME: 15 MINUTES • COOK TIME: 20 MINUTES

Turkey meatballs taste just as good as their beef counterparts but are much leaner, making them a better everyday option. Classic aromatics like onion and garlic powder amplify the authentic meatball flavor. In this twist on sauce that leaves out the tomatoes, a simple garlic and Parmesan sauce coats the noodles and adds complexity in very little time.

FOR THE MEATBALLS

¾ pound lean
   ground turkey
½ cup bread crumbs
1 large egg, beaten
½ teaspoon onion powder
½ teaspoon garlic powder

FOR THE PASTA

8 ounces spaghetti noodles
1 tablespoon
   extra-virgin olive oil
5 garlic cloves, minced
2 cups chopped
   broccoli rabe
¼ cup shredded
   Parmesan cheese
Freshly ground
   black pepper

TO MAKE THE MEATBALLS

1 Heat the oven to 375°F. Line a baking sheet with parchment paper.

2 In a medium bowl, combine the turkey, bread crumbs, egg, onion powder, and garlic powder. Mix well.

3 Shape the turkey mixture into 2-inch round meatballs, and place them on the baking sheet.

4 Bake for 20 minutes, until browned and cooked through, flipping the meatballs once halfway through cooking.

TO MAKE THE PASTA

1 Bring a pot of water to a boil, and cook the noodles al dente. Drain, reserving about 1 cup of the cooking water.

2 In a large skillet, heat the oil over medium-high heat. Add the garlic and cook until fragrant. Add the broccoli rabe and ½ cup of the reserved cooking water to the skillet. Reduce the heat to simmer, cover, and cook for 5 minutes, until the broccoli rabe is fork-tender.

Continued >

Turkey Meatballs and Spaghetti in Garlic Sauce *continued*

3   Add the noodles to the skillet and mix. Add a couple of tablespoons or more of the remaining cooking water to the skillet, to wet the noodles. Stir in the Parmesan cheese and season with pepper. Serve the noodles topped with the meatballs.

Substitution tip: If you don't have bread crumbs on hand, process a piece of white bread, crust removed, in a food processor until finely ground.

Per Serving Calories: 450; Total Fat: 15g; Saturated Fat: 4g; Cholesterol: 100mg; Carbohydrates: 55g; Fiber: 3g; Protein: 23g; Phosphorus: 319mg; Potassium: 354mg; Sodium: 245mg

Marinated Pork Tenderloin

**SERVES 8 • PREP TIME: 10 MINUTES, PLUS 2 HOURS TO MARINATE
COOK TIME: 20 MINUTES**

Pork tenderloin gets credit as a lean cut of meat that is easy to cook right with little effort. This simple marinade locks in the flavor, and searing the meat before roasting it creates a crisp exterior with a juicy, tender interior.

4 tablespoons extra-virgin olive oil, divided

3 garlic cloves, minced

2 tablespoons Dijon mustard

Juice of 2 lemons

1 tablespoon minced fresh thyme leaves

½ teaspoon freshly ground black pepper

2 pounds pork tenderloin

1 In a small bowl, combine 2 tablespoons of olive oil, garlic, mustard, lemon juice, thyme, and pepper. Add the pork tenderloin, cover, refrigerate, and allow to marinate for at least 2 hours or as long as overnight.

2 Preheat the oven to 400°F.

3 In an oven-safe skillet over medium-high heat, heat the remaining 2 tablespoons of olive oil. Remove the tenderloin from the marinade, place in the skillet, and sear on all sides until well browned.

4 Transfer the skillet to the oven and cook for 20 minutes, until the juices run clear. Remove from the oven and cover with foil. Let rest for 10 minutes, cut into ½-inch-thick slices, and serve.

Cooking tip: If you have an instant-read thermometer, use it to check the internal temperature of the pork. It should read 145°F when the meat is cooked.

Per Serving Calories: 192; Total Fat: 9g; Saturated Fat: 2g; Cholesterol: 74mg; Carbohydrates: 2g; Fiber: 0g; Protein: 24g; Phosphorus: 283mg; Potassium: 472mg; Sodium: 151mg

Meatloaf with Mushroom Gravy

SERVES 8 • PREP TIME: 10 MINUTES • COOK TIME: 50 MINUTES

Beef and mushrooms make a complementary duo. Here, cremini mushrooms, also known as baby portobellos or Italian brown mushrooms, elevate the flavor of both the loaf and the gravy.

Nonstick cooking spray

1 tablespoon plus
   1 teaspoon extra-virgin
   olive oil, divided

1 (8-ounce) package sliced
   cremini mushrooms

1 teaspoon dried oregano

1 sweet onion,
   finely chopped

3 garlic cloves, minced

1½ pounds lean
   ground beef

1 large egg

1 slice white bread, pulsed
   in a food processor into
   coarse bread crumbs

¼ teaspoon freshly
   ground black pepper

1 tablespoon
   all-purpose flour

1 cup low-sodium
   beef broth

1 Preheat the oven to 350°F. Coat a loaf pan with nonstick cooking spray.

2 In a large skillet over medium-high heat, heat 1 tablespoon of olive oil. Add the mushrooms and oregano. Cook for 5 minutes, stirring occasionally. Add the onion and garlic, and continue to cook for 5 minutes, until the mushrooms and onion are soft. Remove from the heat. Divide the mushroom mixture into two equal parts, and finely chop one part. Set the other part aside.

3 In a medium bowl, add the chopped-mushroom mixture, beef, egg, bread crumbs, and pepper. Mix well. Form the beef mixture into a loaf and transfer it into the loaf pan. Bake for 45 minutes, until cooked through.

4 In a saucepan over medium-high heat, heat the remaining 1 teaspoon of olive oil, and add the remaining mushroom mixture. Stir in the flour and mix to coat. Slowly add the broth, stirring constantly to break up any clumps. Bring to a boil, reduce the heat, and simmer for 5 minutes, until thickened. Spoon the gravy over slices of meatloaf, and serve.

Nutrition tip: Fresh mushrooms are nearly 90 percent water and are loaded with B vitamins. Low in calories with a meaty taste, they are often paired with beef to lower the calorie count, while adding bulk and flavor.

Per Serving Calories: 280; Total Fat: 20g; Saturated Fat: 7g; Cholesterol: 86mg; Carbohydrates: 7g; Fiber: 1g; Protein: 17g; Phosphorus: 192mg; Potassium: 394mg; Sodium: 146mg

Flank Steak with Chimichurri Sauce

SERVES 6 • PREP TIME: 10 MINUTES • COOK TIME: 15 MINUTES

Chimichurri is an uncooked sauce typically served alongside grilled meats. With Argentinian roots, this sauce works wonderfully alongside a simple flank steak. This recipe uses the broiler for everyday ease, but try cooking the steak on the grill over coals or wood for an even more intense flavor.

FOR THE CHIMICHURRI SAUCE

¼ cup finely chopped fresh parsley

¼ cup finely chopped fresh cilantro

¼ cup finely chopped sweet onion

2 garlic cloves, minced

¼ cup extra-virgin olive oil

2 tablespoons apple cider vinegar

¼ teaspoon freshly ground black pepper

¼ teaspoon red chili flakes

FOR THE STEAK

1½ pounds flank steak

1 teaspoon garlic powder

½ teaspoon dried oregano

Freshly ground black pepper

TO MAKE THE CHIMICHURRI SAUCE

In a bowl, mix the parsley, cilantro, onion, garlic, olive oil, vinegar, pepper, and chili flakes. Use immediately, or transfer to an airtight container and store refrigerated for up to three days.

TO MAKE THE STEAK

1 Preheat the broiler on high. Adjust an oven shelf to be as close to the broiler as possible.

2 Season the flank steak on both sides with the garlic powder, oregano, and pepper.

3 Place the steak on a wire rack over a baking sheet, and cook for 5 minutes on one side. Flip, and cook the other side for an additional 3 to 5 minutes, until desired doneness.

4 Remove from the oven, and tent the steak with a piece of aluminum foil. Let rest for 5 minutes. Slice crosswise against the grain, and serve with the chimichurri sauce.

Substitution tip: For different flavors, you can replace the vinegar with lemon juice, or the cilantro with basil.

Per Serving Calories: 273; Total Fat: 18g; Saturated Fat: 5g; Cholesterol: 77mg; Carbohydrates: 2g; Fiber: 0g; Protein: 24g; Phosphorus: 226mg; Potassium: 416mg; Sodium: 64mg

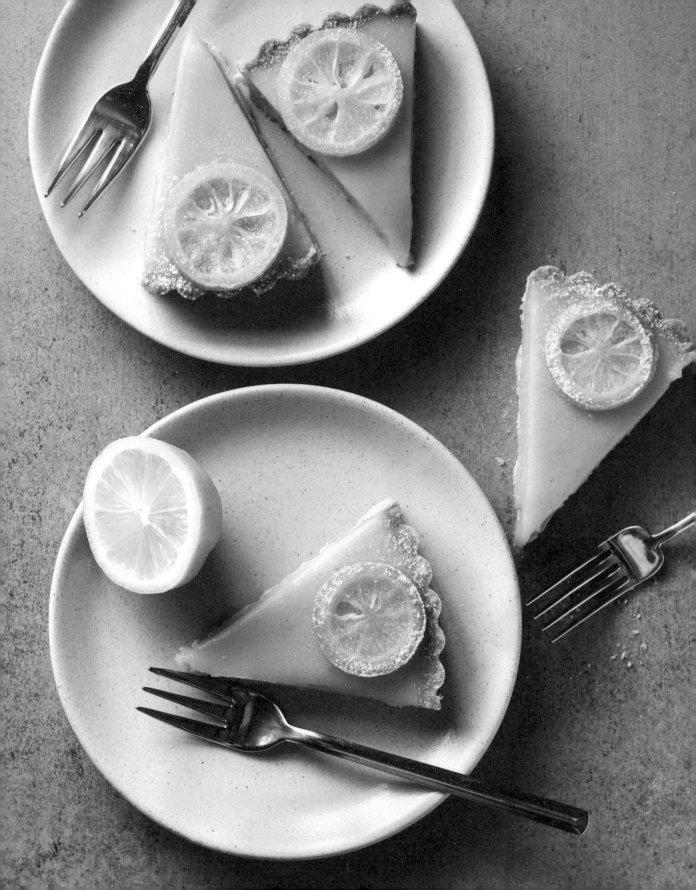

Desserts

◀ *Lemon Tart, page 168*

Tropical Granita

SERVES 4 • PREP TIME: 5 MINUTES, PLUS 2 HOURS TO FREEZE

"Sunshine in a bowl" is a good description for this refreshing dessert. It takes just minutes to pull together before freezing, is perfect for a hot day, and can be endlessly tweaked to suit your tastes. Try this tropical blend and be instantly transported to the Caribbean.

1 cup fresh or frozen
    pineapple chunks
½ cup fresh or frozen
    mango chunks
2 cups orange juice
Juice of 1 lime
Fresh mint, for garnish

1. In a blender, combine the pineapple, mango, orange juice, and lime juice. Process until smooth, and transfer to a freezer-safe dish. Freeze for 2 hours.

2. Use a fork to break the mixture apart into smaller granular pieces. Serve garnished with pieces of torn mint leaves.

Cooking tip: *If you freeze the granita too long, it will become solid. Let it sit out for about 20 minutes until it is breakable, and separate it into a few chunks, then pulse in a blender until its consistency resembles shaved ice.*

Per Serving Calories: 103; Total Fat: 0g; Saturated Fat: 0g; Cholesterol: 0mg; Carbohydrates: 26g; Fiber: 1g; Protein: 1g; Phosphorus: 13mg; Potassium: 145mg; Sodium: 3mg

Grapefruit Sorbet

**SERVES 6 • PREP TIME: 10 MINUTES • COOK TIME: 5 MINUTES
TOTAL TIME: 3 TO 4 HOURS**

Many people say that sorbet can't be done without an ice cream maker, but this recipe proves otherwise. Using just four ingredients, you can create this sweet-and-sour showstopper with just a couple of hours' freezing time. Note: This recipe doubles the amount of simple syrup you'll need. You can refrigerate the remaining syrup to make more sorbet within two weeks.

**FOR THE THYME
SIMPLE SYRUP**

½ cup sugar

¼ cup water

1 fresh thyme sprig

FOR THE SORBET

Juice of 6 pink grapefruit

¼ cup thyme simple syrup

TO MAKE THE THYME SIMPLE SYRUP

In a small saucepan, combine the sugar, water, and thyme. Bring to a boil, turn off the heat, and refrigerate, thyme sprig included, until cold. Strain the thyme sprig from the syrup.

TO MAKE THE SORBET

1 In a blender, combine the grapefruit juice and ¼ cup of simple syrup, and process.

2 Transfer to an airtight container and freeze for 3 to 4 hours, until firm. Serve.

Substitution tip: *Try this with other citrus fruits, such as oranges, lemons, or limes, for an equally delicious treat.*

Per Serving Calories: 109; Total Fat: 0g; Saturated Fat: 0g; Cholesterol: 0mg; Carbohydrates: 26g; Fiber: 0g; Protein: 1g; Phosphorus: 29mg; Potassium: 318mg; Sodium: 2mg

Zesty Shortbread Cookies

**MAKES 16 COOKIES [1 COOKIE = 1 SERVING] • PREP TIME: 10 MINUTES
COOK TIME: 15 MINUTES**

Shortbread cookies are sweet biscuits perfect for eating out of hand or for dipping in tea. They're also surprisingly easy to make from scratch. Using lime and lemon zest enlivens and elevates these simple snappy treats.

1 cup all-purpose flour

½ cup powdered sugar, plus more for shaping cookies

½ cup unsalted butter, cut into ½-inch cubes

Zest of 1 lime

Zest of 1 lemon

1 Preheat the oven to 375°F.

2 In a food processor, add the flour, sugar, butter, and lime and lemon zest. Process until the dough just comes together.

3 Measure a tablespoon of dough, and use your hands to roll it into a ball. Place on a baking sheet, and continue to roll the dough balls until all of the dough is used up.

4 Dip the bottom of a measuring cup into powdered sugar, and press the balls flat with the measuring cup.

5 Bake for 13 to 15 minutes, until the edges are just browned. Transfer the cookies to a wire rack to cool. Store in an airtight container for up to five days.

Cooking tip: You can dust the cookies with a little more powdered sugar after cooking, but while still hot, if desired.

Per Serving Calories: 94; Total Fat: 6g; Saturated Fat: 4g; Cholesterol: 15mg; Carbohydrates: 10g; Fiber: 0g; Protein: 1g; Phosphorus: 10mg; Potassium: 10mg; Sodium: 1mg

Berry Crumble

SERVES 12 • PREP TIME: 5 MINUTES • COOK TIME: 1 HOUR

This crumble customizes with whatever berries you have on hand, making it perfect for cleaning out your freezer and using the last of your seasonal berries. Mix this topping in just minutes, transfer it to the oven, and in a short hour you'll have a dessert to drool over. Let it cool for about 30 minutes to allow the juices to thicken slightly before serving.

6 cups frozen berries (strawberries, raspberries, blueberries, or blackberries)

¼ cup sugar

¾ cup all-purpose flour

¾ cup rolled oats

¼ cup brown sugar

1 teaspoon ground cinnamon

¼ cup unsalted butter, melted

1 Preheat the oven to 375°F.

2 In a large bowl, toss the berries with the sugar. Transfer to a medium baking dish.

3 In the same bowl, add the flour, oats, brown sugar, and cinnamon, and stir well. Pour the melted butter over the mixture, and stir to blend.

4 Using your hands, press the mixture together into pieces, and place the clumps over the berries in the baking dish.

5 Bake for 1 hour, until the top is crisp and browned and the berries are bubbling. Let stand for 30 minutes before serving.

Substitution tip: *You can use pretty much any fruit in a crumble with excellent results. Apples, peaches, pears, and plums also work great.*

Per Serving Calories: 167; Total Fat: 5g; Saturated Fat: 3g; Cholesterol: 10mg; Carbohydrates: 29g; Fiber: 4g; Protein: 3g; Phosphorus: 75mg; Potassium: 155mg; Sodium: 3mg

Grape Skillet Galette

SERVES 6 • PREP TIME: 15 MINUTES, PLUS 2 HOURS TO CHILL • COOK TIME: 25 MINUTES

A galette may sound fancy, but it's simply a rustic pie made in a free-form style. This makes the crust very forgiving, and you don't have to spend a ton of time rolling the dough and working to make it look picture-perfect. With just one bottom crust, folded inward to cover the fillings, the galette looks and tastes great with little effort.

FOR THE CRUST

1 cup all-purpose flour

1 tablespoon sugar

4 tablespoons cold butter, cut into ½-inch cubes

½ cup Homemade Rice Milk (page 70) or unsweetened store-bought rice milk

FOR THE GALETTE

⅓ cup sugar

1 tablespoon cornstarch

2 cups halved seedless grapes

1 egg white

TO MAKE THE CRUST

1 In a food processor, add the flour and sugar, and pulse a few times to mix. Add the butter, and pulse several times until it resembles a coarse meal. Add the rice milk, and mix until the dough starts to come together.

2 Transfer the dough to a clean surface, and shape into a flat disc. Wrap in plastic wrap, and refrigerate for 2 hours or overnight.

TO MAKE THE GALETTE

1 Preheat the oven to 425°F.

2 In a medium bowl, mix the sugar and cornstarch. Add the grapes, tossing to blend.

3 Unwrap the dough and place it on a clean, floured surface. Roll it out into a 14-inch circle and transfer to an oven-safe skillet.

4 Add the grape filling in the center of the dough, spreading it outward, leaving a border of about 2 inches of crust. Fold the edges of the dough inward to partially cover the grapes.

5 Brush the dough with the egg white. Cook for 20 to 25 minutes, until the crust is golden. Let rest for at least 20 minutes before serving.

Cooking tip: *If you don't have an oven-safe skillet, use a large rimmed baking sheet instead. To make cleanup easier, line it with a sheet of parchment paper.*

Per Serving Calories: 172; Total Fat: 6g; Saturated Fat: 4g; Cholesterol: 15mg; Carbohydrates: 27g; Fiber: 1g; Protein: 2g; Phosphorus: 21mg; Potassium: 69mg; Sodium: 65mg

Lemon Tart

SERVES 10 • PREP TIME: 10 MINUTES, PLUS 30 MINUTES TO CHILL
COOK TIME: 30 MINUTES • TOTAL TIME: 3 HOURS, 10 MINUTES

If you're a fan of the lively lemon flavor in desserts, this sweet treat will hit the spot. Because it is rich in butter and sugar, the serving is small, but it packs a giant punch of both sour and sweet that is so pleasing. The no-roll tart shell streamlines prep time and ensures great results every time.

FOR THE TART SHELL

2 tablespoons sugar

1¼ cups all-purpose flour

8 tablespoons unsalted
   butter, melted

FOR THE TART

½ cup freshly squeezed
   lemon juice

Zest of 1 lemon

3 large eggs

½ cup sugar

4 tablespoons butter,
   cut into pieces

1 lemon, sliced, for garnish

Powdered sugar,
   for garnish

TO MAKE THE TART SHELL

1   In a small bowl, whisk the sugar and flour together. Drizzle with the melted butter and stir to blend.

2   Transfer the flour mixture to a tart pan, and use your hands to press the dough to the bottom and sides of the pan. Cover with plastic wrap and refrigerate for 30 minutes.

3   Preheat the oven to 350°F.

4   Prick the tart shell with a fork about 20 times all over, then bake for 20 minutes, until golden brown. Remove from the oven, and cool completely before filling.

TO MAKE THE TART

1   In a medium saucepan over medium-high heat, bring the lemon juice and zest to a boil. Remove the pan from the heat.

2   In a small bowl, whisk the eggs and sugar together. Slowly pour the egg mixture into the lemon juice, whisking constantly. Cook over medium heat, stirring continually, until the mixture has thickened, about 6 to 8 minutes.

3   Add the butter pieces, and remove the pan from the heat. Stir until all the butter melts. Strain the custard through a wire mesh strainer into the tart shell. Refrigerate for about 2 hours, until cold, before serving.

4   Top with the lemon slices and powdered sugar. Serve.

Substitution tip: If you like lemon tart, you can also try the same recipe using limes. Key limes have the most flavor, but the standard grocery-store variety creates a great tart as well.

Per Serving Calories: 252; Total Fat: 15g; Saturated Fat: 5g; Cholesterol: 77mg; Carbohydrates: 25g; Fiber: 1g; Protein: 4g; Phosphorus: 55mg; Potassium: 59mg; Sodium: 29mg

Strawberry Pie

SERVES 8 • PREP TIME: 10 MINUTES • COOK TIME: 20 MINUTES
TOTAL TIME: 3 HOURS, 30 MINUTES

Strawberry pie conjures visions of a summer picnic, and this one's made with a graham cracker–crumb crust, so there is less fat in the final treat than in one made with a traditional piecrust. This is a fresh pie, meaning the strawberries are not cooked, giving the finished product a fresh, straight-from-the-field flavor.

FOR THE CRUST

5 tablespoons
   unsalted butter, at
   room temperature
2 tablespoons sugar
1½ cups graham-
   cracker crumbs

FOR THE PIE

5 cups sliced
   strawberries, divided
¾ cup sugar
3 tablespoons cornstarch
1½ teaspoons
   gelatin powder
1 cup water

TO MAKE THE CRUST

1 Preheat the oven to 375°F. Grease a pie pan.

2 In a small bowl, mix the butter, sugar, and graham-cracker crumbs. Press the mixture into the pie pan.

3 Bake for 10 to 15 minutes, until lightly browned. Remove from the oven and let cool completely.

TO MAKE THE PIE

1 In a small bowl, crush 1 cup of strawberries.

2 In a small saucepan, combine the sugar, cornstarch, gelatin, and water. Bring to a boil, reduce the heat, and simmer until the sauce thickens. Add the cup of crushed strawberries, and simmer for another 5 minutes, until the sauce thickens again. Remove from the heat, and transfer to a bowl. Cool to room temperature.

3 Toss the remaining 4 cups of berries with the sauce to coat, and pour into the pie shell, spreading in an even layer. Refrigerate until cold, about 3 hours, and serve.

Substitution tip: *To save time, you can buy a ready-made graham cracker–crumb crust from the store.*

Per Serving Calories: 265; Total Fat: 9g; Saturated Fat: 5g; Cholesterol: 19mg; Carbohydrates: 45g; Fiber: 3g; Protein: 3g; Phosphorus: 44mg; Potassium: 183mg; Sodium: 143mg

Chocolate Beet Cake

SERVES 12 • PREP TIME: 10 MINUTES • COOK TIME: 50 MINUTES

Beets in chocolate cake? Yes! Beets are a nutritional powerhouse, and while adding them to your dessert may seem strange at first, the beet flavor is nearly undetectable, and all you'll taste is the comforting, chocolaty goodness that chocolate cake is known for.

1 cup sugar

2 cups all-purpose flour

2 teaspoons Phosphorus-Free Baking Powder (page 174)

4 ounces unsweetened chocolate

4 large eggs

¼ cup canola oil

3 cups grated beets

1   Preheat the oven to 325°F. Grease two 8-inch cake pans.

2   In a large bowl, whisk the sugar, flour, and baking powder together. Set aside.

3   Finely chop the chocolate, and melt in a double boiler. Let cool, and mix together with the eggs and oil. Add the wet ingredients to the dry, mixing well to blend. Fold in the beets, and pour the batter into the cake pans.

4   Bake for 40 to 50 minutes, until a knife inserted in the center of the cake comes out clean. Remove from the oven, and let cool. Invert over a plate to remove.

Cooking tip: This cake is great on its own or topped with a bit of whipped cream and fresh berries. Just let the cake cool completely before topping.

Per Serving Calories: 270; Total Fat: 12g; Saturated Fat: 4g; Cholesterol: 70mg; Carbohydrates: 39g; Fiber: 3g; Protein: 6g; Phosphorus: 111mg; Potassium: 299mg; Sodium: 109mg

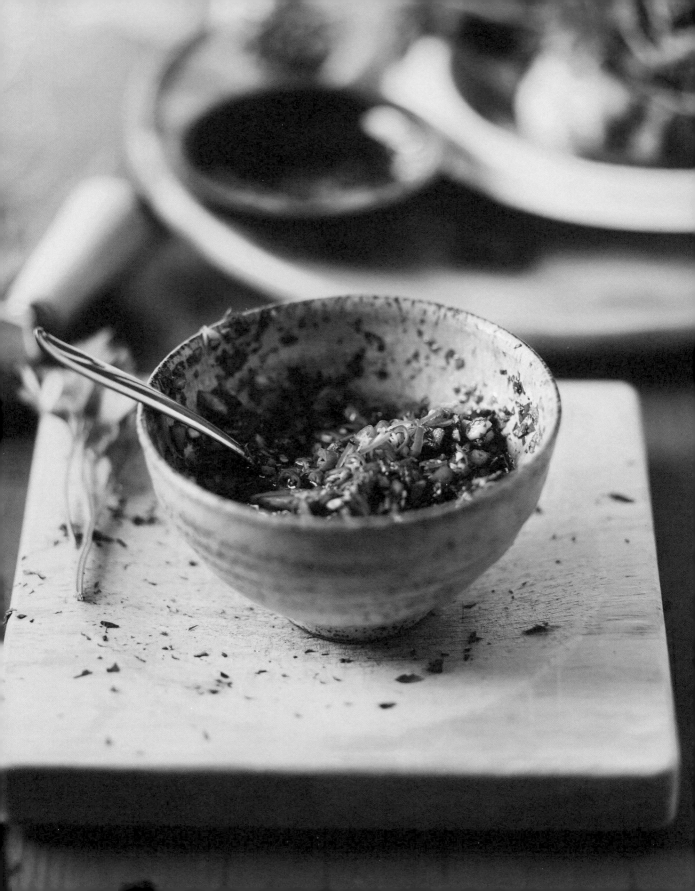

Kitchen Staples

◀ *Balsamic Vinaigrette, page 177*

Phosphorus-Free Baking Powder

MAKES ABOUT ½ CUP [1 TEASPOON = 1 SERVING] • PREP TIME: 5 MINUTES

Baking powder is used in many bread and baking recipes to provide an airy lift. Commercial brands, however, are high in phosphorus, even in small amounts. This quick, phosphorus-free version contains only two ingredients readily available at nearly any grocery store.

6 tablespoons
   cream of tartar

2 tablespoons
   baking soda

Sift the cream of tartar and baking soda together into a small bowl. Transfer to an airtight jar and store in a cool location for up to one month.

Ingredient tip: *Baking soda, or sodium bicarbonate, works as a leavening agent but also has many other uses around the house. It can be helpful in soothing sunburned skin, as a tooth whitener and cleaner, and in various cleaning applications around the house.*

Per Serving Calories: 6; Total Fat: 0g; Saturated Fat: 0g; Cholesterol: 0mg; Carbohydrates: 1g; Fiber: 0g; Protein: 0g; Phosphorus: 0mg; Potassium: 371mg; Sodium: 316mg

Herbs de Provence

MAKES ABOUT ½ CUP [2 TEASPOONS = 1 SERVING] • PREP TIME: 10 MINUTES

Here's a simple spice blend that elevates grilled meats and fish, and adds complex layers to soups and stews. A good all-purpose mixture to always keep on hand.

1 tablespoon
   dried rosemary

1 tablespoon
   dried thyme

1 tablespoon
   dried basil

1 tablespoon
   dried parsley

1 teaspoon
   dried oregano

1 teaspoon
   dried tarragon

In a small bowl, mix the rosemary, thyme, basil, parsley, oregano, and tarragon. Transfer to an airtight container, and store in a cool, dark place for up to one month.

Cooking tip: Herbs de Provence can be rubbed on meats, poultry, and fish before cooking with a little oil to infuse flavor, or it can be added during cooking. It should always be cooked, however, as the raw spice blend can be overwhelming.

Per Serving Calories: 3; Total Fat: 0g; Saturated Fat: 0g; Cholesterol: 0mg; Carbohydrates: 1g; Fiber: 0g; Protein: 0g; Phosphorus: 2mg; Potassium: 19mg; Sodium: 1mg

Cilantro Lime Vinaigrette

MAKES ABOUT ½ CUP [1 TABLESPOON = 1 SERVING] • PREP TIME: 5 MINUTES

This zesty vinaigrette will liven up a salad or marinate a meat with ease. Toss it over mixed salad greens and chopped jicama, or brush it on grilled chicken or steak as it cooks. The cilantro and lime offer bright flavor and color, and this concoction takes only minutes to make, eradicating the need for dubious store-bought dressings.

½ cup packed cilantro leaves and stems

¼ cup extra-virgin olive oil

2 tablespoons freshly squeezed lime juice

Zest of 1 lime

2 tablespoons rice vinegar

2 garlic cloves, minced

¼ teaspoon freshly ground black pepper

In a food processor or blender, purée the cilantro, olive oil, lime juice and zest, rice vinegar, garlic, and pepper. Use immediately, or refrigerate in an airtight container for up to two days.

Substitution tip: Instead of cilantro, this vinaigrette can be made with an equal amount of parsley for a more neutrally flavored vinaigrette.

Per Serving Calories: 50; Total Fat: 5g; Saturated Fat: 1g; Cholesterol: 0mg; Carbohydrates: 1g; Fiber: 0g; Protein: 0g; Phosphorus: 2mg; Potassium: 12mg; Sodium: 1mg

Balsamic Vinaigrette

MAKES ABOUT 1 CUP [1 TABLESPOON = 1 SERVING] • PREP TIME: 5 MINUTES

Knowing how to make a quick balsamic vinaigrette is nothing short of a life skill, especially when you're watching your health. This simple dressing can replace store-bought versions that are high in sodium, sugar, and preservatives. Mix up a batch and use it all week on fresh salads for a quick meal or side—ensuring that you get plenty of vegetables in your diet.

¾ cup extra-virgin olive oil

¼ cup balsamic vinegar

1 teaspoon Dijon mustard

½ teaspoon freshly
　　ground black pepper

In a jar, add the olive oil, balsamic vinegar, mustard, and pepper, and whisk to mix. Store covered in the refrigerator for up to one week.

Substitution tip: This easy vinaigrette can be made with any vinegar you have on hand, but it will taste best if you use a vinegar like apple cider vinegar, rice vinegar, or white or red wine vinegar instead of plain white vinegar, which can be overwhelming on a delicate salad.

Per Serving Calories: 94; Total Fat: 10g; Saturated Fat: 1g; Cholesterol: 0mg; Carbohydrates: 1g; Fiber: 0g; Protein: 0g; Phosphorus: 1mg; Potassium: 6mg; Sodium: 9mg

Creamy Herbed Dressing

MAKES ABOUT 1 CUP [2 TABLESPOONS = 1 SERVING] • PREP TIME: 10 MINUTES

Nearly everyone loves a ranch-style dressing, and this condiment can be especially hard to give up when dieting. And you don't have to with this renal-friendly dressing that shines with the flavor of chives and parsley. Let the cream cheese sit on the counter for a bit before making the dressing to allow for easy whisking, or speed the process with an electric mixer or blender.

¼ cup cream cheese,
   at room temperature
¾ cup Homemade
   Rice Milk (page 70)
   or unsweetened
   store-bought rice milk
1 garlic clove, minced
1 tablespoon chopped
   fresh chives
1 tablespoon chopped
   fresh parsley
Freshly ground
   black pepper

In a small bowl, whisk the cream cheese with the rice milk. Add the garlic, chives, parsley, and pepper, mixing well. Use immediately, or store in an airtight container in the refrigerator for up to three days.

Substitution tip: *This dressing is completely customizable to your tastes. Use oregano, thyme, rosemary, and other household herbs based on what you have available. It's a great reason to grow a small herb garden on your windowsill or outside, so you can reap the health rewards of including fresh herbs in your everyday cooking.*

Per Serving Calories: 57; Total Fat: 3g; Saturated Fat: 1g; Cholesterol: 8mg; Carbohydrates: 7g; Fiber: 0g; Protein: 2g; Phosphorus: 34mg; Potassium: 82mg; Sodium: 37mg

Quick Herb and Oil Marinade

**MAKES ABOUT ¼ CUP [1 TEASPOON = 1 SERVING] • PREP TIME: 10 MINUTES
COOK TIME: 15 MINUTES**

Immerse poultry, meat, or fish in this simple marinade, and then toss it on the grill for a flavorful main dish in minutes. Meat and poultry can marinate just 2 hours to as long as overnight, and fish benefit from 30 minutes to 2 hours.

¼ cup extra-virgin
  olive oil
1 tablespoon red or
  white wine vinegar
1 fresh rosemary sprig,
  leaves only, chopped
2 fresh thyme sprigs,
  leaves only, chopped
3 garlic cloves
Freshly ground
  black pepper

In a small bowl, mix the olive oil, vinegar, rosemary, thyme, garlic, and pepper until blended. Store in an airtight container, refrigerated, for up to three days.

Substitution tip: *Apple cider vinegar can be used in place of wine vinegar. Substitute herbs based on your preferences. Cilantro and parsley are a good replacement for rosemary and thyme.*

Per Serving Calories: 42; Total Fat: 5g; Saturated Fat: 1g; Cholesterol: 0mg; Carbohydrates: 1g; Fiber: 0g; Protein: 0g; Phosphorus: 2mg; Potassium: 7mg; Sodium: 0mg

Simple Chicken Broth

**MAKES ABOUT 8 CUPS BROTH, PLUS 4 TO 5 CUPS CHOPPED MEAT
[1 CUP BROTH = 1 SERVING] • PREP TIME: 10 MINUTES • COOK TIME: 2 HOURS**

Homemade chicken broth is completely doable, and with very little work. This recipe leaves you with several cups of cooked, chopped chicken, as well as a flavorful, sodium-free base useful for soups, stews, sides, and sauces.

1 whole chicken,
   2½ to 3 pounds
1 sweet onion, diced
2 large carrots, diced
2 celery stalks, diced
3 garlic cloves, crushed
1 bay leaf
Freshly ground
   black pepper

1 In a large stockpot, add the chicken and cover it with water. Add the onion, carrots, celery, garlic, and bay leaf. Season generously with pepper.

2 Bring to a boil, reduce the heat, and simmer, covered, for 30 minutes. Skim any residue that forms on the surface. Remove the chicken from the pot, and set it in a colander placed over a bowl to cool. Continue simmering the broth.

3 When the chicken is cool enough to handle, remove the meat from the bones, and return the bones to the pot of broth. Simmer for an additional hour.

4 Meanwhile, transfer the chicken to an airtight container to refrigerate.

5 Strain the broth into small storage containers and let cool for about 30 minutes on the counter. Cover and transfer to the refrigerator.

6 Once cold, remove any fat from the surface of the broth, cover, and return to the refrigerator.

Cooking tip: To simplify your future meal prep, store the chicken in 1- or 2-cup storage containers and the broth in 1-, 2-, or 4-cup containers.

Per Serving Calories: 38; Total Fat: 1g; Saturated Fat: 1g; Cholesterol: 0mg; Carbohydrates: 3g; Fiber: 0g; Protein: 5g; Phosphorus: 72mg; Potassium: 206mg; Sodium: 72mg

Cranberry Ketchup

**MAKES ABOUT 1½ CUPS [1 TABLESPOON = 1 SERVING] • PREP TIME: 5 MINUTES
COOK TIME: 20 MINUTES**

*Fruit ketchups were once plentiful in American kitchens. Today, tomato ketchup
is really the only ketchup around; however, this cranberry version may just
become a staple on your table. It's great on sandwiches, and not surprisingly,
it pairs especially well with turkey as well as beef and pork.*

1 (12-ounce) package fresh
   or frozen cranberries
½ cup chopped
   sweet onion
2 cups water
½ cup apple cider vinegar
½ cup sugar
¼ teaspoon
   ground cinnamon
¼ teaspoon
   ground allspice
¼ teaspoon ground
   mustard seeds
Freshly ground
   black pepper

1 In a small saucepan, add the cranberries, onion, and
water. Bring to a boil, reduce the heat, and simmer,
covered, until the cranberries are softened, about
10 minutes.

2 Remove the pan from the heat, and using an
immersion blender, purée the cranberries. If you don't
have an immersion blender, you can use a traditional
blender, and then return the mixture to the saucepan.

3 Stir in the vinegar, sugar, cinnamon, allspice, mustard
seeds, and pepper, and simmer, uncovered, stirring
regularly, until thickened, 5 to 10 minutes.

*Nutrition tip: Cranberries are a rich source of anti-
oxidants and contain anticarcinogenic properties. The
tannin present in cranberries increases urine acidity
and inhibits bacteria from attaching to the bladder and
urinary tract.*

Per Serving Calories: 25; Total Fat: 0g; Saturated Fat: 0g;
Cholesterol: 0mg; Carbohydrates: 6g; Fiber: 1g; Protein: 0g;
Phosphorus: 3mg; Potassium: 20mg; Sodium: 1mg

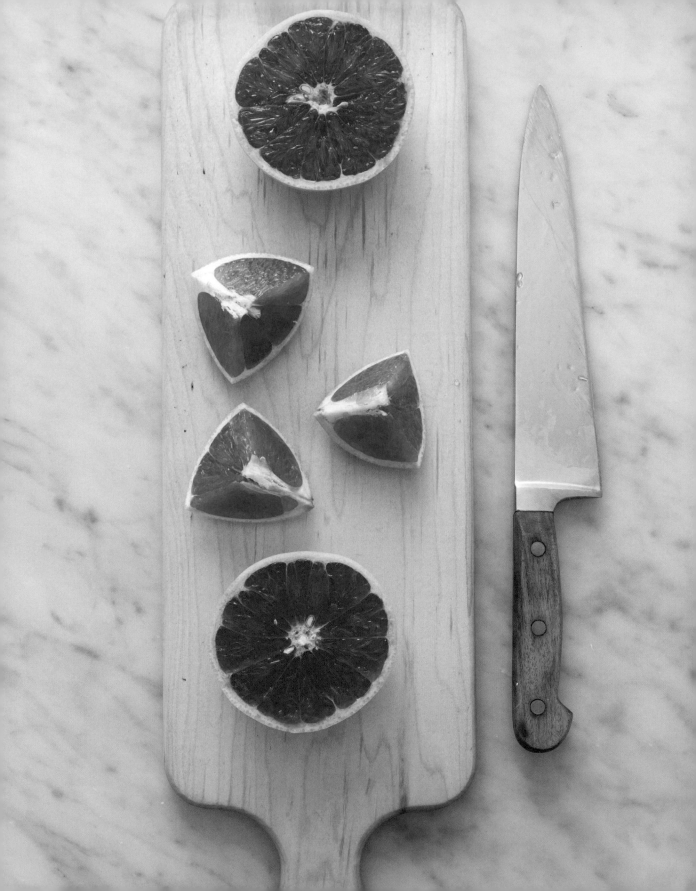

The Dirty Dozen and The Clean Fifteen

A nonprofit and environmental organization called Environmental Working Group (EWG) looks at data supplied by the US Department of Agriculture (USDA) and the Food and Drug Administration (FDA) about pesticide residues and compiles a list each year of the best and worst pesticide loads found in commercial crops. The Dirty Dozen list advises which fruits and vegetables you should always buy organic. The Clean Fifteen list lets you know which produce is considered safe enough, when grown conventionally, to allow you to skip the organics. This does not mean that the Clean Fifteen produce is pesticide-free, though, so wash these fruits and vegetables thoroughly.

These lists change every year, so make sure you look up the most recent before you fill your shopping cart. You'll find the most recent lists as well as a guide to pesticides in produce at EWG.org/FoodNews.

2017 Dirty Dozen		*2017 Clean Fifteen*	
Apples	Sweet bell peppers	Asparagus	Papayas
Celery		Avocados	Pineapples
Cherry tomatoes	In addition to the Dirty Dozen, the EWG added two foods contaminated with highly toxic organophosphate insecticides:	Cabbage	Sweet corn
Cucumbers		Cantaloupe	Sweet peas (frozen)
Grapes		Cauliflower	Sweet potatoes
Nectarines		Eggplant	
Peaches		Grapefruit	
Potatoes	Hot peppers	Kiwis	
Snap peas	Kale/Collard greens	Mangoes	
Spinach		Onions	
Strawberries			

APPENDIX B
Measurements and Conversions

Volume Equivalents (Dry)

US STANDARD	METRIC (APPROX.)
⅛ teaspoon	0.5 mL
¼ teaspoon	1 mL
½ teaspoon	2 mL
¾ teaspoon	4 mL
1 teaspoon	5 mL
1 tablespoon	15 mL
¼ cup	59 mL
⅓ cup	79 mL
½ cup	118 mL
⅔ cup	156 mL
¾ cup	177 mL
1 cup	235 mL
2 cups or 1 pint	475 mL
3 cups	700 mL
4 cups or 1 quart	1 L
½ gallon	2 L
1 gallon	4 L

Volume Equivalents (Liquid)

US STANDARD	US STANDARD (OUNCES)	METRIC (APPROX.)
2 tablespoons	1 fl. oz.	30 mL
¼ cup	2 fl. oz.	60 mL
½ cup	4 fl. oz.	120 mL
1 cup	8 fl. oz.	240 mL
1½ cups	12 fl. oz.	355 mL
2 cups or 1 pint	16 fl. oz.	475 mL
4 cups or 1 quart	32 fl. oz.	1 L
1 gallon	128 fl. oz.	4 L

Oven Temperatures

FAHRENHEIT (F)	CELSIUS (C) (APPROX.)
250°F	120°C
300°F	150°C
325°F	165°C
350°F	180°C
375°F	190°C
400°F	200°C
425°F	220°C
450°F	230°C

Weight Equivalents

US STANDARD	METRIC (APPROX.)
½ ounce	15 g
1 ounce	30 g
2 ounces	60 g
4 ounces	115 g
8 ounces	225 g
12 ounces	340 g
16 ounces or 1 pound	455 g

Resources

Academy of Nutrition and Dietetics: Find an RDN EatRight.org/find-an-expert

American Association of Kidney Patients AAKP.org/support-groups

American Kidney Fund KidneyFund.org

Environmental Working Group: Food Scores EWG.org/foodscores

National Institute of Diabetes and Digestive and Kidney Diseases
NIDDK.nih.gov

National Kidney Foundation Kidney.org/patients

Renal Support Network rsnHope.org

USDA body weight planner/calorie counter SuperTracker.usda.gov/bwp/index.html

USDA food label information ChooseMyPlate.gov/budget-food-label

References

American Dietetic Association. "Pocket Resource for Nutrition Assessment." Accessed June 4, 2017. dpg-storage.s3.amazonaws.com/dhcc/resources/PocketResources /PRNA%202009.pdf.

American Kidney Fund. "Symptoms of Chronic Kidney Disease." Accessed May 15, 2017. www.kidneyfund.org/kidney-disease/chronic-kidney-disease-ckd /?gclid=CjwKEAjwvMnJBRCO2NSu-Puc6AUSJAAf-OSUS8h1dmpXLRS1 onlQXeCLYuLM8NTlPfMhcEHFnRmrLhoCT4Lw_wcB#symptoms.

American Kidney Fund. "Kidney Friendly Diet for CKD." Accessed June 5, 2017. www.kidneyfund.org/kidney-disease/chronic-kidney-disease-ckd /kidney-friendly-diet-for-ckd.html?referrer=https://www.google.com.

Babb, Michelle. *Anti-Inflammatory Eating for a Happy, Healthy Brain.* Seattle: Sasquatch Books, 2016.

Centers for Disease Control and Prevention. "Smoking and Tobacco Use: Fast Facts." Accessed July 24, 2017. www.cdc.gov/tobacco/data_statistics/fact_sheets /fast_facts/index.htm.

DaVita Healthcare Partners. "Dietary Protein and Chronic Kidney Disease." Accessed June 19, 2017. www.davita.com/kidney-disease/diet-and-nutrition/diet-basics /dietary-protein-and-chronic-kidney-disease/e/5302.

DaVita HealthCare Partners. "Glomerular Filtration Rate." Accessed July 24, 2017. www.davita.com/kidney-disease/vocabulary/glomerular-filtration-rate/e/5405.

DaVita HealthCare Partners. "Phosphorus and Chronic Kidney Disease." Accessed June 5, 2017. www.davita.com/kidney-disease/diet-and-nutrition/diet-basics /phosphorus-and-chronic-kidneydisease/e/5306.

DaVita Healthcare Partners. "Renal Vitamins for People on Dialysis." Accessed June 5, 2017. www.davita.com/kidney-disease/diet-and-nutrition/diet-basics /renal-vitamins-for-people-on-dialysis/e/7974.

DaVita Healthcare Partners. "Sodium and Chronic Kidney Disease." Accessed June 5, 2017. www.davita.com/kidney-disease/diet-and-nutrition/diet-basics /sodium-and-chronic-kidney-disease/e/5310.

DaVita Healthcare Partners. "Stages of Chronic Kidney Disease." Accessed May 15, 2017. www.davita.com/kidney-disease/overview/stages-of-kidney-disease.

DaVita Healthcare Partners. "Support Groups for People Living with Kidney Disease." Accessed June 1, 2017. www.davita.com/kidney-disease/overview/living-with-ckd /support-groups-for-people-living-with-kidney-disease/e/4926.

Fairshare CSA Collective. *From Asparagus to Zucchini*. Madison, WI: Madison Area Community Supported Agriculture Coalition, 2004.

Katz, Rebecca. *Clean Soups*. New York: Ten Speed Press, 2016.

The Kidney Foundation of Canada. "Sodium (Salt) and Chronic Kidncy Disease." Accessed June 10, 2017. www.kidney.ca/Document.Doc?id=805.

Kidney & Urology Foundation of America. "High Blood Pressure and Kidney Disease." Accessed June 5, 2017. www.kidneyurology.org/Library/Kidney_Health /High_Blood_Pressure_and _Kidney_Disease.php.

Mayo Foundation for Medical Research and Education. "Chronic Kidney Disease." Accessed May 15, 2017. www.mayoclinic.org/diseases-conditions /chronic-kidney-disease/diagnosis-treatment/treatment/txc-20208292.

Medscape. "Chronic Kidney Disease Treatment and Management." Accessed May 15, 2017. www.emedicine.medscape.com/article/238798-treatment.

National Healthcare Group. "Chronic Disease Management: Managing Diabetes. Eating a Healthy Diet." Accessed July 14, 2017. www.cdm.nhg.com.sg/Diabetes /Pages/Eating-a-healthy-diet.aspx.

National Institute of Diabetes and Digestive and Kidney Diseases. "Food Label Reading: Tips for People with Chronic Kidney Disease." Accessed May 16, 2017. www.niddk.nih.gov/health-information/health-communication-programs /nkdep/a-z/nutrition-food-label/Pages/nutrition-food-label.aspx.

National Institute of Diabetes and Digestive and Kidney Diseases. "Kidney Disease of Diabetes." Accessed June 19, 2017. www.niddk.nih.gov/health-information /health-topics/kidney-disease/kidney-disease-of-diabetes/Pages/facts.aspx.

National Institute of Diabetes and Digestive and Kidney Diseases. "Kidney Disease Statistics for the United States." Accessed May 15, 2017. www.niddk.nih.gov /health-information/health-statistics/kidney-disease.

National Institute of Diabetes and Digestive and Kidney Diseases. "Protein: Tips for People with Chronic Kidney Disease." Accessed June 5, 2017. www.niddk.nih.gov /health-information/health-communication-programs/nkdep/a-z /nutrition-protein/Pages/nutrition-protein.aspx.

National Institute of Diabetes and Digestive and Kidney Diseases. "Your Kidneys and How They Work." Accessed July 18, 2017. www.niddk.nih.gov/health-information /kidney-disease/kidneys-how-they-work.

National Institutes of Health. "Kidney Disease: Early Detection and Treatment." NIH Medline Plus 3, no. 1 (winter 2008): 9–10. Accessed June 19, 2017. www.nlm.nih.gov/medlineplus/magazine/issues/winter08/articles /winter08pg9-10.html.

National Kidney Center. "Chronic Kidney Disease Causes." Accessed May 15, 2017. www.nationalkidneycenter.org/chronic-kidney-disease/causes.

National Kidney Center. "Chronic Kidney Disease Facts." Accessed May 15, 2017. www.nationalkidneycenter.org/chronic-kidney-disease/facts.

National Kidney Disease Education Program. "How to Read a Food Label." Accessed May 16, 2017. www.nutrition.va.gov/docs/UpdatedPatientEd /Lable_Reading_CKD.pdf.

The Renal Association. "Nutrition in CKD." Accessed June 4, 2017. www.renal.org /guidelines/modules /nutrition-in-ckd.

Robinson, Jo. *Eating on the Wild Side*. New York: Little Brown and Company, 2013.

U.S. Food and Drug Administration. "Food Additive Status List." Accessed July 14, 2017. www.fda.gov/food/ingredientspackaginglabeling/foodadditivesingredients/ucm091048.htm.

U.S. National Library of Medicine. "Diet: Chronic Kidney Disease." Accessed May 18, 2017. www.medlineplus.gov/ency/article/002442.htm.

Wood, Rebecca. *The New Whole Foods Encyclopedia*. New York: Penguin, 2010.

Zogheib, Susan. *Renal Diet Cookbook*. Berkeley, CA: Rockridge Press, 2015.

Zogheib, Susan. *Renal Diet Plan and Cookbook*. Berkeley, CA: Rockridge Press, 2017.

Recipe Index

Index

Acknowledgments

I want to thank my Heavenly Father because through Him all things are possible. Thank you, God, for the vision and purpose for this book. Special thanks to my family, sisters, brothers, and friends who contributed words of encouragement.

I would like to thank everyone who helped me complete this book: to all those who provided support, talked through my ideas, read, wrote, offered comments, and assisted in the editing, proofreading, and design. A huge thank you to Stephanie Legin, Patty Consolazio, Katherine Green, and Therezia Alchoufete.

A warm thank you to Clara Song Lee—thank you for trusting in me.

About the Author

SUSAN ZOGHEIB was born in Beirut, Lebanon, and moved to the United States with her family in the late 1980s. She is a registered dietitian (RD) and holds a master's degree in nutrition communication from Ryerson University in Toronto, Ontario. Susan is a leader in the field of renal nutrition, with over 10 years of experience working as a clinical dietitian in various arenas.

Susan is the author of the bestselling *Renal Diet Cookbook* and, more recently, *Renal Diet Plan & Cookbook*: *The Optimal Nutrition Guide to Manage Kidney Disease*. She likes to keep her recipes simple, fun, and full of flavor—and loves to encourage others to get in the kitchen and cook.